A
Personal/Planetary
AWAKENING
Kundalini Style

DBA Spiritual Emergency

Robert Davis MA

ISBN: 1-4392-6439-2
ISBN-13: 9781439264393

This work is dedicated to four of the most loved and cherished people in my life. My two beautiful children Tassa Briel Greif and Braelyn Ayers Davis and the best parents a young soul could have, Robert Davis and Donna Davis.

Thank you for your patience and your love, for allowing me in your life and being in mine.

Love, Robert

Aloha,

It is a time of great change that offers untold opportunities in the fields of self awareness and self healing. The adjustment to this new paradigm is not always easy, yet all have the innate ability to access and benefit from alignment. From the multitude of self imposed constraints sparkles always the light, a light that allows, invites and honors integration and integral confluence. A Personal/Planetary awakening is afoot, a continuum experience that this work touches lightly upon. Numerous pages could be dedicated to the subject of Planetary scenarios, for there are many. I in turn used very few. My casting of the Planetary connection is out of conviction and inklings, sensed and felt to be part and parcel of the whole ball of wax. Though brief it perhaps offers a contextual glimpse into a process that is forever in spiral becomings, sparkling with an eternal knowing, amidst a star strewn backdrop of divine gratitude and grace.

Namaste ala metta.

Robert
Lighttransitions.com

Planetization   1

�֍ �֍ ✖

Chapter I: Planetization

✵ ✵ ✵

Life and death are a snapshot of the continuum of what we call existence: the inbreath and out-breath of being. All existence is in process, in a state of continual emergence.

"Spiritual emergence" constitutes the stage of emergence whereby humankind and all life confront the transformational reality of the Void.

The Void is the outbreath or Shunya (Nothingness) and simply demands complete and total surrender. Innate to Gaia and all king/queendoms of life, this surrender comes naturally, devoid of ego, as a rythmic dance of renewal. Emergence continues through the various stages of life until the periodic death of form.

Through the enrichment of ego and separateness, humans have been buffered in degrees from this natural rite of passage.

Time immemorial is replete with individual transformational occurrences. Most occurred under the auspices of a sacred shamanic process, while others were perhaps relegated to a diagnosis of insanity and dealt with accordingly. This natural transformational process is reflective of the integrational system of planetary evolution and is, in accordance, gaining momentum as we approach the continual and necessary transfiguration of all life. Vedic, theosphical, and anthroposo-phical scholars have all illuminated the periodic transformation of cultural evolution. Hyperborean, Polarean, Lemurian, Atlantean, and present-day cultures are aligned in a spiralic geometric, refle-ctive of both past experience and future potenti-als. As our subtle bodies become truly informed of the evolutionary shift, we become physiologically sensitive, experiencing, in a variety of ways, what is termed Spiritual Emergency(A multi dimensional physiological crisis).

Planetization and the process of integrati-onal becoming have grown acute due to the shift in dimensional activity from one paradigm, or Meme, to another, i.e., the fourth to the fifth dimension.

I. History of Evolutionary Axial Periods

The play of continual unfolding has burgeoned at specific times in our history. This I liken to axial phases from which emerge defined chreodes, or potential paths, of evolutionary possibility: 600-450 B.C. and 1855-1955 A.D. are two such periods. These catalytic epochs were cosmic propellants serving as enhancements to the planet along its spiralic path, hastening its development as if an evolutionary light had been infused into the Planet's noosphere or etheric field. Humankind's shift from viral to positive symbiont is the balancing result; 600-450 B.C. witnessed post-Atlantean caty-lists such as Lao Tsu, Buddha, Socrates, Mahavira,

Confucius, and the epic Bhagavad Gita. This period amplified the unity paradigm of this cycle in its nascent stage and served as precursor to the very pregnant axial phase of 1855-1955, which has seeded the present stage of planetary emergence, resulting in a spectrum of transformative emergings and openings. This will unfold in parallel to the increase in temporal reality as vibration heightens and physical reality adjusts to a new, unified plane of being.

The speed of the unfolding is relative to the individual. Simply stated, it is achievable not on the plane of its conception but on a plane of its realization. That plane of realization has become more accessible as more individuals access and attune to its definition. The definition is individualized via access and blooms into a universalism by attunement. Attunement is a byproduct, not a procurement, of process, and is unique to each individual. Unity and universalism scent and color the individual's plane of realization, evoking a co-sharedness of life, until differentiation fades into the mist of universal connectivity.

Spiral Pathways into the Mist

The Earth has and will continue to go through transformative stages — as have all living things. There have been innumerable catastrophic occurrences in the Earth's past, many of which have gone unrecorded in the exoteric sciences; however, the intuitive arts are clear on the sacred transference of culture amidst dramatic earthly changes. The spiralic pathway of esoteric antiquities casts a multidimensional light on heritage and human potentials, illuminating future/present sciences in the field of healing, medicine, architecture, and energy.

Spiritual energy has demonstrated guidance via inter-and intra-dimensional stimulus, such as individualized guides, crop circles, extraterrestrial contact, and spiritual teachings. The emergence/emergency process we are now experiencing has roots dating back hundreds of thousands of years on Earth, as on other planets.

For our purposes, we are going to briefly look at two previously mentioned epochs of time, 600-450 B.C. and 1855-1955 A.D., with soul influences that are thought to be axial periods of stimulus prestaging the present unity consciousness emergence.

600-450 B.C. Post-Atlantean Era

Seedings of energy are necessary to catalyze and co-create the life force impulse, which, through the higher laws of discernment and optimization, gropes eternally for fullfilment; 600-450 B.C. resonates with a special frequency of unity direction. Soulful sparks were amplified and intoned with a unificational theme. Buddha, Lao-tzu, Confucious, Mahavira, Socrates and the archetypal Bhagavad Gita infused the cultural energy with witness identification and the interconnectivity of all life. This theme has always been true and accessible; however, the 600-450 B.C. seeding reflects a pulse that soon quickens in the sense of Cosmic time. The pulse sounds out the frequency and laws that are refined and eventually integrated into form.

We, as a planet and culture, are going through a transfiguration that is refective of the amplified messaging of the 600-450 B.C. pulse. Our transfiguration is of an organic nature and is receptive to many multidimensional inputs, in addition to the physical plane stimulators. This nexus of time is, of course, part of a continuum of time and energy, representing infinity in its befores and afters. After the last stage of Atlantis (10,500 B.C.), with the submergence of the final island remnant, we find a stream of informational transference leading first to ancient India and the Manu in the Himalayas, the creation of the Vedas, and, later, the Upanishads, and on to the antiquital Egyptians with the construction of the pyramids and Sphinx. Rama, Thoth, Hermes Trismegistus, Krishna, and Zoroaster all appeared and were light contributors before Lao Tsu, Buddha, Mahavira, Socrates and Confucius. The key to the axis of 600-450 B.C. was the illumination of global consciousness on the Eastern part of the planet on a physical plane. It was a time of enlivening, like a germ spot on an egg.

II. Apexual Relevance to Current Epoch

What emerged was a unity consciousness that, in its nascent stage, was cradled in the most socially active part of the planet. It was the springboard of global consciousness and a synthesizer of the illumination predating it, one that reverberates during our current, highly reflective period of individual and global transformation. Pythagoras, Chuang Tzu, Mencius, Meng Tzu, Plato, and Aristotle all contributed to the evolution of consciousness as the cosmic ray of planetary activity moved from East to West with the advent of Jesus and, later, Muhammed.

1855-1955 A.D. Post-Atlantean Emergence

This phase is plethoric with illuminational souls (Chreode Blazers ie,those that forge new ways of being and pathways of living) and serves as a multi-planed stream of evolutionary energy that dynamically organizes and accentuates the pre-required pathways of eminent planetary transformation.

The transcendental poets — Thoreau, Emerson, and Whitman, along with Dickenson — heralded a re-amplification of Light cast upon the emergent culture. The Theosophical founders — Leadbetter, Blavatsky, Judge, Olcott, and Besant — westernized ancient Indian teachings and, along with Rudolph Steiner (through anthroposophy), provided accounts of antiquital cultures that stretch the empirical time continuum into necessary expanded dimensions.

The westernization and globalization of spiritual evolution has been sparked, leading toward the next (spiralic) level. As this transcended and expanded history is disseminated, a grand current of Indian teachers are set aflow from East to West: Meher Baba, Sai Baba, Osho, Swami Satchidananda, Neem Karoli Baba, Hazrat Inayat Khan, Pir Vilayat, Sri Yukteswar, Baba Hari Dass, Aghoreshwar Baba Bhagwan Ramji, Sri Aurobindo, Sri Swami Rama, Swami Vivekananda, Mishio Kushi, George Osawa, Paramahansa Yogananda, Thich Nhat Hahn, Maharishi Mahesh Yogi, Swami Sivananda, Krishnamurti, Sri Rama Krishna, A.C. Bhaktivedanta Swami Prabhupada, Swami Mutkananda, Ammachi, Darshan Singh, Sri Ramana Maharshi, Sri Poonjaji, and Swami Vivekananda; and Western-Easteners such as Da Free John, Ram Dass, Satguru Sivaya, Subramuniyaswami, Sri Kriyananda and Gangaji.

Others who have contributed to the expansion of planetary potentials and chreodes in the light of a new transformational paradigm include: The Huxley family (Aldous, Julian and Thomas), Margaret Meade, John Todd, Dr. Seuss, Carlos Castenada, Isaac Asimov, Robert Heinlein, Arthur Clarke, Linus Pauling, Peggy Omera, H.G. Wells, Stephen Hawkins, John Mitchell, Stanley Kubrick, Linus Pauling, Fritzof Capra, Mother Teresa, Bill Surtleff, Eckert Tolle, Stephen Gaskin,

Louis Leakey, Stephen Spielburg, Immanuel Velikovsky, Albert Einstein, Samuel Clemens, Coleman Barks, Sir Arthur Conan Doyle, George Lucas, James Lovelock, Lester Brown, Stewart Brand, Michael Jacobsen, Paul Erlich, Lewis Mumford, Buckminster Fuller, Arnold Toynbee, William Reich, Arthur Lovejoy, Alfred North Whitehead, Rod Serling, Will and Ariel Durant, Timothy Leary, Werner Erhard, Sir Darwin Gross, Albert Hoffman, Brooke Medicine Eagle, Barbara Marx Hubbard, Rowenee Patee, Jean Shinoa Bolding, Wilhelm Reich, Neil Armstrong, Amory and Hunter Lovins, John F. and Bobby Kennedy, Martin Luther King, Corretta Scott King, George Leonard, Christopher Hills, Howard and Eugene Odum, Gary Snyder, Michael McClure, Lawrence Ferlinghetti, Bob Dylan, Allen Ginsberg, Al Walford, Billy Graham, Bob Keeshan, Mr. Rogers, Stanley Krippner, Marilyn Ferguson, Stanislav Grof, Nelson Mandela, Lech Walesa, Anita Roderick, Peter and Eileen Caddy, Edgar Cayce, William Irwin Thompson, Gregory Bateson, Wayne Dyer, John Lily, Elizabeth Kubler Ross, Steven Levine, Hazel Henderson, Loren Eiseley, Gabriel Roth, Jacques Cousteau, Ralph Nader, Dennis Kucinich, Kurt Vonnegut, Dennis Hayes, Alice Walker, Doris Lessing, Rupert Sheldrake, Paolo Soleri, Roy Eugene Davis, Helen and Scott Nearing, Murshid Samuel Lewis, Pierre Teilhard de Chardin, Ken Keyes, Jr., Thomas Edison, Nikolas Tesla, Gurdjieff and P.D. Ouspensky, Rachel Carson, Aurelio Peccei,

Jeramy Rifkin, John Robbins, Bob Marley, The Beatles, John Mack, Alice Bailey, Michael Jacobson, William James, Carl Jung, Oswald Spengler, Martin Buber, Stanislav Grof, Houston Smith, Ken Wilbur, Henry Bergson, Richard Bucke, Ignatius Donnelly, William McDonough, Paul Hawken, David Zink, Herman Hesse, Frank Herbert, E.F. Schumacher, Alberto Vilardo, J.R.R. Tolkein, Alvin Toffler, Alfred North Whitehead, Peter Tompkins, Amory Lovins, Alex Grey, Stephen Schwartz, Desmond Tutu, Dalai Lama, Brian Swimme, Marshall Mcluhan, Joanna Macy, Ivan Illich, Carlos Castaneda, Al Gore, Hazel Henderson, Rupert Sheldrake, James Redfield, Luther Burbank, Alister Crowley, Gustav Holst, Albert Einstein, Deepak Chopra, T.S. Elliot, Terrence Mckenna, Jean Houston, Ralph Abraham, Kahlil Gibran, Alvin Toffler, John Lily, Michael Murphy, Ignatius Donnelly, Jose Arguelles, Francis Morre Lappe, Riane Eisler and Albert Hofmann.

The visible, manifest characteristics are numerous and varied: crop circles, Auroville, Arcosanti, dolphin and whale communication, greenhouse effect, Earth Day, increases in ET abductions and DNA human/ET research and acknowledgments, Findhorn, The New Alchemy Institute, World Watch Institute, Rocky Mountain Institute, Buckminster Fuller Institute, Intentional Community Network and Eco Village training center at the Farm, Abode of the Message, Dmanhur, Esalen Institute, and Omega Institute. Key media include: *What* the Bleep, One Giant Leap, Ayurveda: The Art of Being, Waking Life, The Secret, ET, and Close Encounters of the Third Kind, as well as key books: On Walden Pond, Leaves of Grass, The Essays of Ralph Waldo Emerson, The Secret Doctrine, The Urantia Teachings, Cosmic Memory, Life and Teachings of the Masters of the Far East, Ohaspe, The Book of Secrets, Autobiography of a Yogi, The Diamond in Your Pocket, The Population Bomb, Silent Spring and Diet for a Small Planet.

Chapter II: My Story

✵ ✵ ✵

Emergence has been on my mind for many, many years, knowing as I do that the primary goal of my life was to transcend ego and reach a point termed "enlightenment." However, this concept was elusive in its practical employment. It seemed a world apart from the collective sense of life I had known. As if on a clock, the transcendent sirens beckoned me to come home.

I started to sense the unity of all life in 1977, when I was twenty-four. I had lived a full, beautiful life up to that point. My parents, Robert and Donna, were and are archetypes of grace and caring. They were there for me always, caring for me in sickness and supporting my visions in health. My challenges as an only child and young person were few; however, I did experience illness. I had encephalitus (theoretically) three times and almost died at four months old. According to my mother, had it not been for the holy water sprinkled on my "limp" body, I probably would have died. She claims I smiled; I cannot remember.

I was also exposed to a babysitter who spared no details in recounting metaphysical stories about hauntings and spiritual visitation. These experiences frightened me and catalyzed a tendency in me to wet the bed as a young child, which I eventually outgrew.

I went on to experience grade school in Muncie, Indiana, and in Indianapolis (where we moved in 1962). I enjoyed my junior and senior high school years, playing basketball and baseball religiously.

In my senior year, I was confronted with a very powerful experience. At a party, a friend asked if I wanted to try the Ouija board and I accepted. I was informed as to the process and the purpose, as well as how to touch the plachet and use it as an interdimensional tool for contacting the dead.

"Well," I said, "let's check on Jimi Hendrix" (since he had just passed on).

"Sure," was the reply and we were off.

Immediately, as we touched the plachet, it began to move smoothly and purposefully, spelling out a "yes" to affirm that we were in contact with Jimi Hendrix.

Fascinated, I asked something like, "How is it wherever you are?" and the reply was, "It is good, very good."

Feeling a little more self-assured, we ventured on to contact one of our classmates, who had died recently in a plane accident. When we asked more about his death, the contactee detailed how the altimeters and plane equipment gauges failed, and I sensed we had found a tool for multidimensional communication. Neither I nor my friend were versed on plane equipment gauges.

The evening went on with other people "playing the board," focusing on dating questions and light party fare. My friend and I sensed that the board wanted us for more. We later decided to set up a time to explore the board and the connections it afforded us in depth.

Our exploratory started at John's house one afternoon after school. I asked the board who we were in contact with and it answered, "Joseph, of Joseph and Mary." Then the plachet started to move at an abnormal rate of speed, with both of our hands attached to it. As it moved from letter to letter, we quickly realized it had a biblical energetic. We later looked up the message and found it to be a quote from the Bible.

At other sessions, because of the speed of the plachet, we had to enlist a reader to write down the letters. This process led me to start hearing voices and seeing doves at timely intervals. I started carrying a small Bible and felt connected to something I had no answer for.

One afternoon, John and I set a Bible down beside us on the floor and lit a candle. Joseph started to speak through the board and said I was to be a fisher of men and that there were seven planes of existence. Additionally, he said there were going to be twelve major communities at the time of change and that I was to be intimately involved with one of them. I said that

I was a bit afraid of the path laid out for me and the board answered,"Robert, look to thy left foot and, John, look to thy right foot, and ye shall be healed." John and I simultaneously looked down at our respective feet and found the Bible.

After that message, I heard something fly from the porch, and the plachet on the board immediately stopped. I asked, "Are we still in contact with Joseph?" The board answered, "Nay, Joseph left with the flight of the dove."

Then the plachet took off and kept spelling, "I am a damned spirit, I am a damned spirit" over and over. The candle at our feet burned very high and intensely. We gladly called it a day.

From that point on, things are a little fuzzy, except that I remember we brought in some Jesuit priests for observation. They had no directional advice and served in the capacity of witnesses. Over the three or so months of this adventure, I became open to a new intuitiveness, along with hearing voices. I finally had to burn the board when I started getting touched lightly on the head at night. The net result was that I had tapped into some subtle plane of energetic existence outside of the conventional plane paradigm.

I remember asking Joseph, vis a vis the board, "Why contact me through the board?" The answer was, "Because this was the only way you would hear it." I did hear it and it remains discernible as an early opening point to the multidimensional existence of energy and life.

Concurrent to this time, John and I developed an amazing sense of clairvoyant telepathy between us, being able to guess written numbers in the five- to six-digit category. This telepathic connection seemed to parallel our mutual involvement with the Ouija board and ended after our experimentation.

After high school, I went on to four undergraduate and two graduate schools. I only touched the Ouija board one other time and that was at MacMurray College in my freshman year. A friend wanted to talk to his deceased mother so I suggested the Ouija board. I watched as he contacted what he wanted to believe was his mother then broke down emotionally as a result. From that point on, I left the Ouija board to others so inclined.

After MacMurray College, I went to Indiana University-Purdue University in Indianapolis, St. Petersburg Junior College (Clearwater campus), and University of Florida, where I graduated with a bachelors degree in political science. One of the highlights while attending the University of Florida was witnessing a talk by Howard and Eugene Odum, Gary Snyder, Allen Ginsburg, and Michael McClure on "Steady State" energy systems. I was drawn to the energy modeling of the Odum brothers, particularly their energy flow diagrams. It made sense to me poetically, like a lyrically transcendent song.

Two souls that impacted my life in Gainseville were Robert and Pia. Robert was a wisened Socratic-style friend/teacher who showed me the art of evaluational thought and subsequent conscious action. Pia was a beautiful sparkle from Sweden. She embodied a feminine self-assurance that touched me deeply. Her self-assurance and self-knowledge became traits I sought out in all of my future relationships. I have not heard from nor seen either of them in thirty-one years. I loved them both.

After the University of Florida, I was hired by TWA as a flight attendant and moved to New York, before getting laid off. I then drove to California with my girlfriend, whom I met in the latter part of my senior year at the University of Florida. I worked in San Francisco as an order book official at the Pacific Stock Exchange and a commodities option broker. Neither job agreed with my temperament due to my growing sensitivity to ethics, greed and money. My girlfriend and I drove back East, both realizing it was time for us to go our separate ways. I dropped her off in Pennsylvania and went back to my parents' home in Marlton, New Jersey. I took various jobs to offset my expenses to my parents: assistant manager of store detectives at a department store, school bus driver for a private school, and a warehouse dock worker.

At this time, I started what seemed to be an emergence in the sense of intuiting positive planetary futures. I became fascinated with solar homes, alternative energy, and positive global evolution. I would go to visit earth-sheltered homes designed by Malcolm Wells and read extensively about steady state planetary existence.

The Club of Rome and Buckminster Fuller's World Games primed my interest in being an active participant in the positive unfolding of the planet. I decided to go to the University of Maryland and get my MA in urban planning and community design. It was 1977. Off to college again I went. I drove down to Hyattsville from Marlton, New Jersey, in a U-Haul equipped with enough furniture for a small house.

After staying in a short-term rental outside the beltway, I found a nice duplex and began looking for three roommates. Two out of three were involved with Eckankar, and I was exposed for the first time to a vegetarian diet. My interests in solar energy and self-sufficiency blossomed.

Graduate school at the University of Maryland was known to some degree as a feeder system into HUD (the office of Housing and Urban Development). I was interested in community design and development and would have had to pursue a dual degree in architecture. Although that is appealing now, at the time I was becoming more interested in the energetic element of community design from alternative energy to the quality of human existence within the community. This concept of qualitative human existence touched me deeply and was amplified by my reading the works of Lewis Mumford. *The City in History* and *The Story of Utopias* set me on a path of discerning qualitative options for the pathway of human evolution. I was drawn to the Yes bookstore in Georgetown and began a cosmic readathon, directed by instinct and divine providence. My perception of time and space was changing as I was led to the works of Pierre Tielhard de Chardin.

Reading most of de Chardin's work, I became convinced that we, as a culture, were evolving spiritually at a quickened pace and that the design of future communities must take into account the evolving human spirit as well as a symbiotic relationship with the planet. I was able to get credit at the University of Maryland for an apprentice job at the Institute for Local Self-Reliance. My job was to help design and build a demo solar hot water heater at the institute. (I still have the drawings.)

The landscape around me lightened even as Reagan dug into the White House and negated the National Center For Appropriate Technology. I saw for the first time the energy of polarities, whereby a Darkness affords an equal balancing effect of Light. I started working for love at the Solar Energy Institute and orchestrated the first Sun Games held on Washington Monument grounds in May of 1978.

Esoteric literature fell off the shelves into my eager hands at the Yes bookstore: Edgar Cayce and ARE, *Life and Teachings of the Masters of the Far East*, *The Aquarian Gospel of Jesus the Christ*, *The Urantia Teachings*, *Dweller on Two Planets*, *Oahspe*, *The Secret Doctrine*, every written book I could find on Atlantis and Lemuria to books by and about Rudolf Steiner, who became a pivitol piece of my soon-to-emerge thesis. I felt a surge of global transformation all around me as, book by book, I was led into an information base that would fuel my thesis and guide me to a plane of clear thought that afforded me insight into what I believed was an emergent culture.

I felt that cultural transformation was a consistent part of our cosmic past and would continue into the cosmic future. After Lewis Mumford, Arnold Toynbee, a newly acquired vegetarian diet, and an avalanche of esoteric cosmic literature, I was no longer fit for the University of Maryland.

So, despite my 3.0 GPA at the University of Maryland, I sought out Goddard for its flexibility and structure as an institution. I met with the core faculty advisor and was on my way.

My next step was to define what I wanted to pursue, so I stated my focus as planetary development, along with cosmosgenisis, anthropogenisis, and spiritual evolution. My two ground theorists were Pierre Teilhard de Chardin and Rudolf Steiner (de Chardin provided an empirical slant to justify spiritual evolution in humans, whereas Steiner povided a cosmic time tree of events spiraling back beyond exoteric time scales). I used Steiner's cosmic time tree as a road upon which my thesis traveled. I needed a field faculty advisor so I asked the president of the Solar Energy Institute.

He agreed and I moved to Washington, Virginia, where I lived for a year in what was called the White House. A two-hundred-year-old home, bordering the Blue Ridge National Park, the house had no running water or bathroom. I had a wood cook stove downstairs and a tin stove in my room, which taught me to appreciate a quick, hot fire. This was my thesis-writing abode and the first place I had ever lived where the silence had a sound — and it was loud.

The process involved periodic trips into D.C. (eighty miles away) every couple of weeks to check in with my faculty advisors. I worked a little at the Solar Energy Institute and gave required talks on planetization.

I also went to Plainfield, Vermont, for colloquims on several occasions and had wonderful encounters. Several of my graduating classmates were involved in related fields. One was studying ley energy line configurations in England and another was studying color therapy. I remember a tall, white-haired man from Brazil who was a core faculty advisor in that country. He had a special radiance about him and was familiar with Pierre Tielhard de Chardin. He sought me out and asked me to come to Brazil to study. I was tempted but was compelled to stay in my program, with its existing structure.

I left that particular colloquium feeling connected to my path and grateful for the connections I had made. One friend gave me a picture of the Sphinx he had taken in Egypt on the evening he spent a night in the queen's chamber of the Great Pyramid. I still have that photo hanging in my living room.

The year I spent in Washington, Virginia, was a period of intimate involvement with Pierre Teilhard de Chardin and Rudolf Steiner. I fashioned a wooden altar from a fallen tree to write upon. I spent some time with the East Coast Rainbow family tribe and was deeply appreciative of their friendship.

The White House had a graveyard on the north side, surrounded by a rock wall. I remember coming home late one evening and parking about a half mile from the house. As my dog Cody and I approached the house, I was stopped cold by the energetic display of lightning bugs on the maple in the middle of the graveyard. They were pulsing from the ground up through the leaves in rythmic patterns. That image remains a visual tattoo from my time at the White House. Another event during my stay there involved the seven-year locust. I got up one morning and heard an incredible sound, a sound that I would attribute to a large UFO. The pitch and intensity drew me outside, where I encountered a hillside of locust-covered apple trees. I immediately walked up the hill into their midst and felt as though I were being bathed energetically with a frequency from another dimension. The volume and depth of the sound remains with me still.

As my thesis evolved, my appreciation for the White House grew. Originally it was a segue home into the Washington, Virginia, community. Then it became a launch pad, leading me to tofu making.

My journey from the White House and the Washington D.C. area was mixed with joy and sadness. I was leaving many friends and a major transformative space in my life. Cody by my side, I left with a large bag of fresh peaches and headed off to Indiana to attend my grandfather's funeral.

When I got to Muncie it was wonderful to see my parents and grandmother, as well as my cousins. After the service, my cousin Saddhen asked me to come down to Bloomington, where he had started a tofu shop called Simply Soyfoods.

Loving both tofu and adventure, I went, explaining to my parents that I would meet them in St. Louis after a brief visit to Bloomington.

Once there, I was ushered into Saddhen's shop under The Gabels restaurant and was overwhelmed with familiarity. I sensed I had made tofu before and knew, upon walking into Simply Soyfoods, that I would make it again. The water, the smell, the positive energy and love all beckoned, as did the taste of fresh tofu with a dash of Dr. Bronner's mineral boullion and the freshly made Tofu Spicey Joe. Dharma (purpose) looked me in the eye and I blinked.

That evening, Saddhen and I went out to eat then spent time on the roof of his house, talking about life and tofu. The next evening we visited a friend of his, who believed in the concept of tofu making. He gave my cousin and me the money to start Light Foods in St. Louis. I remember leaving his house and seeing a shooting star — and I knew it was magically meant to be.

The next day, I left Bloomington to go to St. Louis, Missouri, to stay with my parents as I searched for just the right location to start a tofu shop. It took me about six months to locate the right spot, incorporate, bring in some investment, piecemeal some equipment together, order more equipment from Japan, and learn how to make tofu again.

Bill Shurleff's book, *The Book of Tofu and Soymilk Production,* was indespensible. It was the tofu bible of the mid- to late-1970s. Bill brought tofu into consciousness in North America. For the first several months, my mother and I made all the tofu and cleaned up afterwards, often putting in eighteen-hour days. I remember we got the tofu account for the Soycrafters Conference in Urbana, Illinois, in 1980. We worked for what seemed like three days straight to produce 1,000 to 1,200 pounds of tofu.

We soon brought in employees, and I was in a complete state of gratitude and appreciation. My mother and father were both vital to the establishment of the company. My mother worked physically with me, as well as being the bookeeper at the shop, and my father helped with costing all the products I invented, as well as offering his astute business insight. My mother did her fair share of inventing as well (Atlantean Marinade, Donna's Deva cookies and The Pies in the Skies). It was such a time of blessing that stood out as pivitol to my understanding of Dharma.

One morning, I got up (I lived in an apartment right above the tofu shop) and cried for about an hour, knowing deep within that I was exactly where I was supposed to be at exactly the right time. I started my days at 3:00 A.M., when I would get up, grab my dog, and drive over to Forest Park, where I would run three to four miles. I would come home, do yoga, sit quietly for a while, take a shower then go down and start the boiler, clean the equipment, grind the first batch of beans, cook the 'go,' press out the okara, and fix my first glass of steaming fresh soymilk on my way to grabbing the nigari pail (to use in coagulating the first batch of tofu). My goal was to have seven batches in process before the morning crew came in at around 8 to 8:30 A.M. I usually hit my goal.

Light Foods was about selling Light; the food was secondary. My mother, Donna, was the cornerstone of the enterprise. We marketed tofu and secondary soyfood products (soysage, soyloaf, tofu cream pies, pot pies, whipped tofu cream, fruit butter frozen cookies, marinated tofu, etc.) to the Midwest regional market.

It was at this time in 1980 that I started working on soy ice creams with Bailey Farm Dairy in St. Louis. We were almost ready to start marketing pasturized soy milk and ice cream when the opportunity arose to develop a tofu hot dog. As a result, the first tofu hotdog was born: Light Links. I set up national, natural food distribution within a few months and unveiled it in New Orleans at a Natural Foods Show in the summer of 1982.

Al Jacobsen, who started the Garden of Eaten, came up to me and said, "Congratulations. I knew somebody was going to do it." It happened because I wanted to get tofu into the mainstream of thought and diet, and the hotdog trojan horse was an avenue.

✳ ✳ ✳

I got married in 1981 and my life changed. My first child, Pir, died after one day from a respiratory distress syndrome via Beta strep. The event spawned years of poetry as a means of processing. (The mourning reached a stage of completion only recently.)

In 1983, I decided to focus on meat analogs, i.e., tofu hotdogs (Light Links), tofu baloney (Light Loney), Soysage, tofu sausages(Tofu Browners), the first Tofu Bagel Dog, etc. Consequently, I sold the tofu equipment and moved to California to work with a series of meat packers (Made Rite Meats, which went Chapter 11, and Safeway in Stockton). My wife and I found a beautiful home and and energetic town in Nevada City, California. Safeway produced the bulk of my products at that time, through 1989. The years in Nevada City and Grass Valley were blessed in that they brought two beautiful, brilliant children, Tassa Briel Davis, in 1985, and Braelyn Ayers Davis, in 1987, into our lives. My life felt full and blessed.

In 1989, we decided we wanted to be near water and a Waldorf school, so we searched and found Whidbey Island in the Puget Sound. Off we went to Whidbey Island, where I started Believe Inc. (the first organic based soy and rice ice cream) in 1990. Concurrent with this, Light Foods went into Chapter 11 and I went through a divorce.

The great pain of not being with my children full-time was difficult to process and I became dedicated to part-time parenting as much as humanly possible. My children were the light in my life and have remained so. My prayers would always start with asking for the ability to take care of and be involved with my children. My prayers were answered because I worked from home and was almost always able to take them to school and pick them up, and to be there for their special events. I was graced in the enactment of my prayer.

My goal was to stay on the island and co-parent my children, which necessitated a great deal of business creativity, leading to the following companies and positions: the establishment of Ecotrition Foods, a sub-company of Believe, which focused on meat analogs like the Bounty Burger and The Eco Burger, along with a list of meat-style soy-based products, all packed for Food Service. I worked as a consultant to my friend Yves on his Burger Burger product in 1992, and with my friend Richard on the Hemp Rella and Vegan Rella alternative cheese line in 1993.

I started Savin Grace, an organic cotton/hemp naturally-dyed clothing company in 1993, and worked with Sunfeather Herbal soap company. I lifted one- and two-man rocks between jobs for about four months in 1997 then worked with Good Karma foods to 2008 (which developed Soy Dream Ice Cream and Organic Rice Divine). I have been trying, since my initial opening when I was twenty-seven, to fully allow my heart and passion an audience, via a right livelihood/business. I have infused many projects and jobs with my passion, always waiting for the service opportunity matched to my heart, soul, and Dharma.

I wish blessings on all my endeavors and work-related associates, in that I have learned much from each of them.

Chapter III: Personal Evolution of Process

✳ ✳ ✳

The start of my 'energetic process' was in 1993, after my divorce and the loss of my business, Believe Inc./Ecotrition foods. I developed (theoretical) prostatitis, had some night sweats and went through a few weeks of dark night soul-dancing. Through it all, I wanted to stay on the island because of my love for my children.

So the job loss and divorce settled into my body and became a mysterious allopathic disturbance. I remember my allopathic doctor intuitively touching my chest above my heart and bringing tears to my eyes. He then said I needed to get some bodywork. I appreciated his sense, even though he put me on a month-long regimen of antibiotics. Later, I went to a more alternative physician and, over time, the condition cleared up — yet, until recently, never completely went away.

I changed employment and was left to dance again with the dark night of the soul. My ailment came back, this time with more of a chronic fatigue, flushing, hot hands, and symptoms of Epstein Barr. Moving on to a naturopath, I went along the homeopathic, moderately energetic pathway, yet no one to date said I should see a transpersonal psychologist or psychiatrist. It was still a dimensionally locked approach with some aromatherapy and emotional tinctures thrown into the mix. I came out of round two around 1996.

The next dark night came in 1997 after another change of career, and left me with no alternative but to start working on the island as a laborer in construction landscaping. I would often trail behind a back hoe, where I would lift one-man and two-man rocks into place. It was humbling and humorous, finding myself, at forty-four, with a masters degree and years of alternative business experience doing what felt like prison labor; however, it provided the balance I needed to write a children's story titled *The Star Children*.

I reached a point where I was down to, literally, my last dime and was ready to jump on my bike and start riding down I-5 South to somewhere, when an old friend called and asked if I would develop a rice alternative cheese for him and his company. I did so and this was the start of my time with Good Karma Foods.

In 2000, I moved into a chemically toxic house and took another energetic hit. This episode rekindled the chronic fatigue and left me seeking an emotional reset in my own home with just my children. In retrospect, this time was more about my imminent opening than temporal circumstantial components. I knew deeply that a time was coming when I would reach the edge of reality and functionality. But I needed to be available to help my children through high school and I was. Through this period, both of my children extended compassion and understanding to me. My daughter, Tassa, was on her own and experiencing the world of Seattle, while my son, Braelyn, was enjoying his high school years with me.

The years 2003 to 2005 were a staging period; first I had a herniated disc in my neck then, in 2004, my energetic restructuring started to apex (chronic fatigue, altered psychology, insomnia, ideated suicide). Lastly, from January to November of 2006, came the orgasm of fear, God, and dual realities.

The Disc

The herniated disc came from a running accident I had in the fall of 2003. I was running down a hill on a paved road and my right shoelace caught on the tread of my left shoe and displaced my feet from the road, resulting in a headfirst fall. I threw out my arms to break my fall, allowing me to go into a left shoulder roll. Intense shock to my neck caused the hernia at C3 C4, but only after I was bike riding and taking pictures with a thirty-pound backpack strapped to my back in Port Townsend. When I got home that evening, I was a little stiff; on waking in the morning, I found I could not move my body because of the pain.

Three to four weeks of muscle relaxers, oxyco-done, and some prednisone left me a bit imbalanced. I was fast on to an allopathic mechanical fix.

Slowly, I recovered. Physical therapy twice a week helped some but it was time, and the suggested procedure of a spinal fuse, that gave me focus.

As spring of 2004 unfolded, I was biking ten miles a day and running two, drinking two or three soy lattes, a little champagne and playing ping pong after a fifteen-mile ride — and I felt good and tired. My son was heading into his junior year, attentive to his surroundings and his quality time in high school.

In the early summer of 2005, my son and I went through several car crashes involving his Subaru WRX; there were no physial injuries but a lot of stress and energy loss. This started the last phase of intensification, spanning the next two years. My body was in a theoretical stage five adrenal burnout, which was assessed via a hair mineral analysis. I had intense heat, on-the-clock flushing, extreme fatigue, and insomnia.

So I shifted to the most progressive alternative clinic in the Northwest and went through nearly two years of alternative treatment based on Lyme disease, mercury poisoning, mold toxicity, weakened adrenals, parasites, liver and kidney disfunction, etc. I had just about every test. The catchall was adrenal insufficiency and toxic overloads.

I received energy adjustments at times via one of the clinic's physician bodyworkers and noticed results. My primary doctor was an angel, a blessing and very well intentioned. However, everyone was after the holy grail of physical answers, including me. I knew something was coming, but could not identify the process.

Slowly I made my way through the evolutionary diagnostic stream, relieved each time that I would find an answer, only to see my energy shapeshift into another symptom and new frontier. I was wearing down and preparing for the orgasmic period.of total breakdown and surrender.

The intensification was fast approaching along with the new year (starting with Christmas of 2005). I knew it would be my last year as a householding parent, though it was an honor watching my last child graduate.

I noticed a very small scab on my left cheek that would not fully heal. It had bled and healed over a number of times, so I decided to take matters into my own hands. I knew of a product called Black Salve, a historic anticancer cream. I went on the Internet and researched it as best I could. My dermatologist was gone for the holidays and I was anxious to address the issue. I called my naturopath and had them rush-deliver Black Salve to me. As if by divine providence, it appeared at my doorstep the next morning. From that expedience, I assessed that 'spirit' wanted me to use the Black Salve.

That evening, Christmas Eve, I put a pea-sized piece of salve on the scab and covered it with a small, round band-aid. The next morning the spot enlarged to the size of a nickel and the following day to the size of a quarter.

Looking to the Internet for reassurance (since no one was available to consult), I felt somewhat calmed by the testimonials I read about healing and scarring. Nevertheless, I was a bit concerned about the speed and size of the forming scab, with which a strong, painful stinging was associated.

After three days, I knew this would take me into another dimension of physical self-worth and ego. I knew this meant that it was time for me to face things. I was ready, or so I thought.

By the time a week had passed, a plug the size of a quarter, about a half-inch deep, started to emerge from my left cheek. On New Year's Day, the scab came out, leavinng a cavernous hole in the left side of my face. Stunned and yet okay with the experience, I rested in the confidence that it would heal perfectly with a moderate trace of scarring.

As the months passed, the incomplete healing of my cheek accompanied my declining health and emotional imbalance. Amidst the decline, I had my work to contend with, along with the joy and emotional pain of my son's last months with me at home. I had to hold on and I did, by a thread.

☆ ☆ ☆

The intensity of my job and the traveling to a cold climate on four separate business trips, between February and May 2006, left me drained and weakened. The first trip in February brought on a 104-degree fever my first night in the hotel and lasted for twenty hours.

The intensity of the stress and the environment over the next three trips eroded the energetic outer shell of my resistance. By the time the end of May came around, I could go no further without a diagnosis. I underwent a battery of tests (including an MRI and a CAT scan), saw a cardiologist, and mainlined costly Glutathione. I was also getting acupuncture from a gracious Eastern healer to whom I would often go to for help or to use her spare healing room as a safe haven.

Living became intense, as I spent a lot of time on the acupuncturist's floor, shaking and wanting to die.

My reality started to split in two. One was my former reality, in which everything was in place, and the other was a different dimension, where life as I had known it did not exist. It was a world of disenfranchisement, isolation and separatism. Once there, I could not access my former space and time of linear logic and comfort.

I still had to hold on and make it through a planetary war of Saturn and Mars, plus my current astrological cycle of Sade Sati (when Saturn transits your natal moon). I also had to attend my son's graduation and maintain the connection with my former wife.

The apex of the planetary war arrived. As I sat at my son's graduation, heat started to flow uncomfortably through my body and I felt my face redden as I endured being in the auditorium with all of the other parents and the graduates. I took pictures of my son as best I could and made it to his graduation party, hosted by Braelyn's girlfriend's parents (who were angelic to Braelyn and me).

After the party, I went straight to the acupuncturist's office, finding a room and a floor to sit on. My doctor was a very good person who went out of her way to help me. Acupuncture and energy work seemed to balance me for two to three hours, sometimes longer.

Now that my son had graduated and I had met with my former wife, I was ready. I had been told for over a year that I was toxic, so I hit the low PH diet for several weeks and planned to visit my friend and go through a Pancha Karma (which manifested into a Kaya Kalpa procedure). So off I went to California at the end of June 2006 (barely able to walk) to stay with my friend and go through the cleansing.

My friend lived next to a graveyard in a beautiful town. The area I had visited years ago now took on a shaded, alternative reality. I was picked up at the Oakland Airport in the afternoon and taken to an ashram. The orginal plan for a Pancha Karma shifted because of the Vedic practitioner's reluctance to treat me in my condition. So a secondary plan evolved for me to see an ayurvedic doctor who practised an esoteric branch of cleansing called Kaya Kalpa. I had to wait several days to meet the doctor and his wife due to appointment schedules.

I went to the ashram, altered and physically depleted. I was dropped off in the early evening, went to the main office and was shown my room. Everything around me was differentiated and separate. I was there in my room on the floor, feeling the peace, yet feeling hopeless about ever regaining what I thought was normalcy.

There was a cooling breeze that evening, which helped because I could hardly walk amidst the challenges of orientating to a new place. My friend returned later to take me to someone who was skilled in the art form of jin shin jitsu, a gentle point activation energy work system analogous to finger-activated acupunture. It, like accupuncture, brought me back to fifty percent of my energetic, which was amazing and vital.

Enlivened a bit, I went back to the ashram and tried to sleep. I had been on high-test, natural sleep aids for five months because of severe insomnia. Again I popped the pills and caught my usual five to six hours, waking before dawn a bit groggy and wondering, "Where am I, and where am I going?"

I was still limited to my walking range of about 100 yards (I had been a runner for thirty years, averaging two to three miles a day), so I wandered around the ashram briefly, trying as always to associate with some aspect of my former life. Satisfied, I did a bit of yoga and meditation. I went into the community kitchen and fixed myself a nutbutter sandwich and decided it would be an okay place to die. I felt relieved that I could die someplace away from my children and not put them through an immediate trauma.

The guru arrived the second day from Seattle. When I was introduced to him, he looked at me deeply and asked, "Where is Robert?" I could not answer, only knowing I was clearly nowhere.

While going through the treatment, my house on Whidbey was being boxed up and painted inside and out for a sale. Now that my son had graduated, it was my time to move. Little did I know at that instant that the prophesied movement was to be mostly internal.

My talk with the guru revealed a connection that manifested when his assistant asked me to look at a residence that was soon to be available at the ashram. I had been in contact with a divine psychic throughout my journey so I called her for an opinion on this residence. She said it was evident that, through trust, my path would become manifest. Incidentally, that was exactly what the guru had told me earlier in the day, and no doubt what I would have told myself had I asked.

So there I was at the ashram, running at about twenty-five percent of my life force, waiting for my friend's space to clear and my appointment with the ayurvedic doctor, which was moved up because of my condition.

My room at the ashram was poolside, so I looked for the most comfortable chair to sit in; there it was in the corner with a foot stool. I was sitting for about forty-five minutes when a kindly soul walked by me several times. Finally, on the third pass, he asked me if I could move because that was the guru's chair. Of course, I said yes and moved, noting that the chair was without a doubt the one to sit in when out by the pool.

The second evening was comfortable and the food was always wonderful, especially since the guru was back. My friend came over and helped prepare the evening meal.

I felt like I was visiting a movie set as an extra who was chronically ill and dying. The temperature in Sonoma was starting to heat up again and even with a small fan, the ashram room was very warm. Dusk became night. I took my sleeping pills and laid down, wondering how my son and daughter were going to do without me.

Wednesday came and brought with it the move to my friend's place and my five-hour introductory appointment with the Indian doctor. We took off north to Healdsburg, California, to meet with the ayurvedic doctor. Driving through Healdsburg, we went through a subdivision and veered off up a hilly road to the end, where a large, somewhat foreboding brown house stood. We pulled into the driveway and I looked around, feeling a poignant "Where am I?" We got out of the car and went up the steps.

A knock on the door brought a beautiful Kaphaesque woman in her early forties to the door. She was the doctor's assistant and wife, who cordially invited me in, where I was asked to sit and fill out an ayurvedic questionnaire that would reveal my constitution and weaknesses.

I told her I only had $2,500 for the program and hoped it would be enough. She assured me that it would be. (Later, however, I found out it wasn't.) After filling out the form, I was asked to urinate into a clear cup and bring it back to the table.

The doctor, who was responsible for introducing my friend to ayurveda many years ago, came out and sat down to my right. He was sixty-something, exuded a vital energy and looked the picture of health. He looked over my answers and the urine then began his assessment and discussed his protocol. He said I had a Vatta imbalance. My constitution was Vatta Pitta with a lot of Ama (toxicity both emotional and physical); Vatta is Air and Pitta is Fire. The third constitution is Kapha (Water).

Ayurveda is a great integrational system based on thousands of years of practice. Yet my condition was clearly assessed as one with an emphasis on physical Dhatu cleansing. I was up for anything and was still under the impression that I was toxic and loaded with mercury, molds, and allergins. In my mind, all of this was because I was dying, had no immune system, and had chronic fatigue. So I was ready to get clean no matter what, even though I had a hard time walking a block and was having extreme flushing periods.

After the doctor's assessment, we got started. I was led to a rear room, where there was a heated bed with clean white sheets. The windows were drawn and there was a peaceful atmosphere in the room. There was a stereo and a steam cabinet as well. I undressed per his assistant's request and lay on the bed under the blankets. I was then administered some eye and nose drops. I was asked to start breathing deeply through my nose while clenching my sphincter muscle on the inhale and releasing the clenched muscle on the outbreath.

Meanwhile, the stereo played classical Indian ragas and chants. It held three or four CDs, so I heard the same music several times per session.

Next, the doctor came in to join his wife and start administering the herbal paste to the back side of my body. I had to lie stomach down with blankets covering my pasted back until it dried. His wife told me this was the Indian equivalent of a CAT scan and would reveal the level of toxicity present in my body. If the paste turned dark or black, it meant I was toxic. I think mine was pretty dark, or at least it looked dark as I tried to check it out my-self.

As I waited for the paste to dry, I was continuously reminded to focus on my breathing. This was difficult because the bed was nice and warm and I was always tired due to insomnia. Occasionally, I drifted off to sleep and was awakened softly with the request for me to be attentive to my breathing. Meanwhile, the chant music played on.

After about an hour, the doctor and his wife returned to check the paste. When they agreed it had dried, they both started at a foot and worked up my back side, firmly rubbing off the dried paste. Once it was removed, they rubbed in some cleansing oil.

With the back done, they asked me to turn over and applied paste to my entire front side and face. When they finished, I lay back down, was covered, and asked to continue my breathing. This was the first of six cleansing treatments that were to be followed by six rejuvenative treatments. The psychic and my dear friend felt I would only need six or seven treatments. I was not sure how many I would live through.

So, after the front side dried and I had been breathing and listening to chant music for another hour, in came the doctor and his wife to check the paste. Satisfied that it was dry, they duplicated the back process by removing the paste firmly, working up from my feet. They spent a lot of time on my feet and hands when administering the oil.

After that, they had me sit up and poured warm oil on my crown chakra and, for the first three sessions, down both ear canals. With a towel wrapped around my oiled head and slick as a whistle, I was off to the oil-scented steamer cabinet.

The first time I went in, they had it very hot and I thought I had to tough it out. After about fifteen minutes at inferno temperatures and losing what felt like a half gallon of sweat, I melted out of the cabinet and hobbled over to the bed.

Once there, I was prepared for the cleansing enema. The doctor donned rubber gloves then held up a bladder of warm herbal milk admixture. In it went and then I was asked to do a bicycle-type motion to draw the enema high up into my colon. Once it was securely inside, I was led into the bathroom, where a very warm bathtub was awaiting me.

Submerged into the hot water, I was instructed on a pranayama breathing technique to accompany my soaking session. The right to left nostril breathing practice was familiar to me, but was not what I felt like doing at that time. The doctor's wife instructed me the entire first session in breathing: hold a long time then out through the opposite nostril, again and again, until I could hardly hold my arms up to close my nostrils.

Then it was time to expel the cleansing enema. The concept is to force the toxins into the intestine via bodywork and steam then flush them out with the enema. After the evacuation, I was asked to get back into the tub and wait.

The doctor came in with a large container of lukewarm, oily water, which he poured into a dispensing vessel directly above my head. With earplugs in and a warm towel over my eyes, I was ready for the pineal drizzle. The flow was mainly focused on my third eye with intermittent attention to my throat and heart chakras. The breathing was "ah ha ah" on the in and "ha" on the out with some speed consistency.

After about five minutes, my arms started tingling and I felt faint. I was asked to stop the breathing and shift to a slower nose breath. By this time I was barely holding on to reality. The drizzle continued until the vessel above my head was empty. The doctor's wife then came in, washed my hair and rinsed me off. My arms were shaking, and I was very weak and uncomfortable.

I was walked to the bed, where I lay down. She asked me to lie with my arms outstretched, hands open. The energy was so strong I could not keep my palms open, and my fingers were drawn into a fist position. I was told this condition, known as kundalini, would pass.

✲ ✲ ✲

I was grateful that my friend was waiting to drive me back to her house. She was heartful and honorable throughout my travail.

Back in Sonoma, it was starting to warm up into the hundreds with no air conditioning. I was still running hot and flushing, so the temperature was a challenge as I tried to rest. I inadvertently took a powerful herbal sleeping pill one afternoon at the house and the ensuing hours were a struggle to stay awake.

The ayurvedic treatments were $500 each, two to three days apart, depending on everyone's schedule and energy. Traditionally, these treatments were administered in a retreat setting, where the patient would be sequestered between treatments in a closed birthing hut without any external stimulus. I can attest to the need for this as a prerequisite to the process. I, however, was cut loose back into the world into a very safe but hot house next to a graveyard, over an hour away from the treatment center.

The distance was okay until I had to drive myself to the last four of eight treatments. Each subsequent treatment was similar, except the seventh and eighth ones, which were restorative treatments and had a variant enema. The first six were to clear or cleanse the dhatus (tissues), plasma, blood, flesh, fat, bone, marrow, and sexual fluids. That accomplished, I could start with a clean slate and replenish my system for six more treatments.

However, I could only afford three weeks and eight treatments. After treatment number five, I felt close to death, so I asked my friend to take me to the hospital emergency room. The counter energetic to this condition is that I was, and am still, going through Sade Sati, which is a very transformative period, along with a Vedic Dasha sequence that tested my heart and soul.

My friend, being an astrologer, was seeing things clearly from her perspective and a great deal of what I was experiencing was noted in my chart. **This is an important point and one I wish to explore via the connection between Sade Sati and planetary placements in Vedic astrology, with emergence-type phenomena.**

Clearly, in my case, there was a strong correlation. What remained in the final analysis, however, was the question: How do I get through it?

Chapter IV: Flash Point

✵ ✵ ✵

My trip to the emergency room was part of a destined process. I had been leaning toward this experience for months, filled with trepidation as to what would be uncovered.

I was sure that, on this day, someone would discover the answer to my daunting fatigue and unbearable psychological condition. I was prepared to call my children and employer and tell them I was finally diagnosed with "xy" and "z."

In the lobby of the emergency room, I was grateful for what looked like a short wait. Trying to hold on until I was admitted, I scanned the room for other emergency cases, noticing a person with a swollen face and another who was perhaps in for a check-up. Nothing too bad.

Finally, my name was called and I was led to a table for evaluation. With a deep breath, I told the nurse that I thought I was dying of something. We went over the symptoms of flushing, exhaustion, dizziness, metal toxicity, chronic fatigue, Epstein Barr, Lyme disease, mold poisoning, etc. It was a challenge for me to even walk.

The nurse hooked me up to a vital signs gizmo where I was sure evidence of my imminent demise would soon appear. Steadying myself for the quick unplug and whisk into the IC ward, I saw the nurse glance up at the reading and heard her say that everything looked perfect.

How could that be? I thought. *The equipment must need to be recalibrated or the nurse doesn't know how to read it.*

The nurse then said that another nurse would be right down for my blood draw. *Well,* I said to myself, *if it didn't show up on the vitals, my death march will come clean in the blood work.* How could it not in light of how I felt?

My friend left at this point to do some errands and said she would return in just a bit. Before the primary ER nurse left, I asked if he could do some endocronological evaluations. I knew, based on all of my cutting-edge naturopathic evaluations, that my endocrine system was blown.

"Well," he said, "they would go for key indicators and that would alert them to further pathways of exploration if needed."

Okay, I thought, this will be a series of tests, then. The first would tip them off to some tremendous imbalance then they would follow up with the in-depth analytical test that will tell them how long I had to live.

An hour or so passed and my friend came in to check on me. The doctor was now in the general area, reading tests and x-rays for other ER patients. Finally, I got up and walked to the larger office next to my room and asked the doctor how the tests were coming. He said they should be back any time.

I noticed the nurse bringing the doctor some paperwork and he looked my way. *Ah-ha*, I thought, *he is contemplating how to tell me how much time I have before I die.*

He looked over several sheets, laid them down, and walked out of the room. I assumed he probably did not have the nerve to tell me at the moment, so I asked the nurse if those were my blood results. She looked at them and said, "Yes."

Then she looked me in the eye and continued: "Your blood work looks great."

I sat down on the bedside as the doctor came in. "Well," he announced, "everything looks to be in order."

"Order?" I repeated. "I feel like I can hardly walk."

He took a deep breath and asked if I had seen a therapist or psychologist.

"No," I responded. "Why should I?"

"Well, a lot of these symptoms can be psychosomatic."

He was the first physician in my two and a half years of physical decline to mention a therapist. From that point on, it was on the screen, especially as I left to go back to the house by the graveyard.

Many mornings found me at my friend's door filled with a hopeless energy. My friend kept insisting I would eventually get better. On the deepest level, I agreed.

✴ ✴ ✴

The jin shin jitsu worker was a wonderful balancing force throughout the treatments. I would recommend such a course along with Kaya Kalpa or any type of cleansing process. Of course, the service is only complete with a safe house, free of worldly external connection.

I continued on with my cleansing and reached treatment number six, the turning point of my two replenishment sessions. I remember deeply questioning my last two appointments, even though they were "restorative."

The culmination of my cleansing would come with my friend's imminent departure to the Midwest. After treatment seven, I started anticipating my own move back to Seattle. The destination was bursting with loss and alternative realities: no place to live, my daughter's cancer screening surgery (cone biopsy), my father's prostate cancer treatment, and my dear friend's supposed stroke.

With psychic counseling and my friend's encouragement, I went for session eight. There was a new assistant at the ayurvedic doctor's house who would be helping during my session that day. As I was waiting in the living room, I heard the doctor talking to this person (who had worked with him in Los Angeles). He was explaining my case to her and alluded to the theory that I had a mental problem.

This caught me a bit off guard and I went into the kitchen where they were conversing and said, "You can come out here and talk about this if you need to."

This caught them by surprise and the assistant came out to the living room to hear my explanation.

I said, "My daughter is having a cervical cancer screening operation, my father is undergoing radiation treatments for prostate cancer, I have no place to live and my best friend has just had a theoretical stroke" (which was later found not to have been a stroke). I added, "And, by the way, I can hardly walk and feel like I am dying."

She looked at me a bit stunned and with compassion, which I welcomed. But now it was time for treatment number eight. In I went, hoping that my second rejuvenative treatment would reverse what felt like a downward spiral of energy and attitude. Knowing that I was to board a plane in two days — to return to an empty house and a circumstantial nightmare — made me hopeful for the miracle of feeling better.

The treatment ended and I had my customary, gourmet, ghee-laden Indian soup then said my heartfelt goodbyes to the doctor and his wife while packing away a month's supply of ayurvedic herbs.

The drive back to my friend's home was particularly difficult that day. Traffic was slow and the temperature was hot. I must say that I am not drawn to go back to Nothern California again in this lifetime, but I will always honor the gracious heart of my friend and the astute perceptions and blessings of the guru at the ashram.

✳ ✳ ✳

The flight back to Seattle conjured feelings of fear and confusion. My friend, who was going to pick me up, could not because of the theoretical stroke he'd had, so his wife's brother appeared at the airport to drive me to the ferry.

My daughter had asked me to attend her operation, but I could not because of my exhaustion. It was with a very heavy heart that I made my way to the Whidbey Island ferry, where I was dropped off, carrying my two heavy bags.

I felt very weakened and totally overwhelmed by my daughter's condition, my father's radiation treatments, my friend's theoretical stroke, and my homeless state.

The sun was shining as the ferry crossed the water (it was August). I felt relief coming back home, but to what?

My surroundings started to take on a surreal quality as we approached my past life and my home, in a new, altered state. Pulling up in the driveway, I could see that my former home had been painted and looked mortuary-friendly. My friend said she had found a place for me to stay and that my former house was too toxic for me to sleep in.

Once out of the car, I started calling out for my disenfranchised cats, both of whom had been on the lam for the last three weeks. Food was provided for them during this period by my son, his girlfriend, and her wonderful parents. The cats, however, were rarely seen and came in to eat through a cracked rear door. I was hopeful they would remember my distinct cat call, and they both did eventually show up. I could not stay with them long, though, bound for another unknown residence.

I petted them and told them I would return, but wanted to take my daughter's cat to honor her pre-op request. I walked into what was once my home and felt alone and frightened. Every element that represented my life was gone or altered. The house had been completely repainted inside and out and every personal item was packed up and placed in the garage. My son had directed the process while I was in Sonoma. It was a quick growth period for him and he adapted to it with grace and responsibility.

As I looked around in my weakened state, I felt that it was indeed a time of total loss and I had no idea how I was going to make it through the fire of this experience. The house was toxic on many levels, so I decided to go with my friend.

When we arrived at the home of another friend, who I only knew marginally, I took my bags out of the car and carried them inside, set-ting them down in the living room, where I was to sleep. Thoughts of my imminent demise flooded my soul as I sat down in the living room, bewilde-red and shocked as to how abruptly my life had disintegrated into a freefall of physiological fai-lings and personal loss. Sade Sati, transformation, and potential death stalked me relentlessly. But the pastoral setting suited my immediate need for tranquility and safe surroundings, however discon-nected to my reality they were.

The owner of the home was kind and generous and was available for periodic chats and check-ins. I found this process helpful in that it allowed me to verbalize my perspective and drain the toxic pus of confusion, fear, and death.

I still used a natural sleep aid and rarely slept longer than four to five hours, usually waking be-fore dawn. This period was always difficult in that it allowed a free swing of amplified, discordant thought that resulted in a deepening depression.

At the first light, I would attempt a few exercises (sit-ups and push-ups) and yoga before walking a paltry block. I was always trying to reconnect to my exercise routine, which had been a great part of me and was now just a poor shadow-refection.

After my walk, I would fix an egg with some miso/tahini toast and tea, refraining from coffee, which I had quit several months earlier. This routine lasted for about a week until I realized I could no longer sleep in this kind person's living room.

On a Sunday, I got up and went over to my former home and packed up some of my daughter's belongings, as well as some of mine, then took off to live with my daughter in Seattle. Tassa, while recovering from her biopsy, offered me heartful assistance through a difficult situation. In the back of my mind, I knew Seattle would be a much more accessible location to medical assistance, because I knew deeply that I would be needing it.

Before moving, I tried to secure antidepressants through a local Whidbey Island psychiatric nurse, who told me she was not taking any more clients but recommended Lexapro at 10 mg per dose, if I could get it. I then called my naturopathic doctor, who called in the prescription.

Off I went to Seattle with my Lexapro in hand. When I got there, I drove to my daughter's work location in Ballard, where she was employed as a barista.

She was waiting outside the coffee shop with a smile, to direct me to available parking. I remember how tired I was walking to meet her and how grateful I was to see her.

Once inside, I mentioned that I needed to see a psychiatrist so she looked through the yellow pages and wrote down about ten names. I chose Dr. David because he was located about one mile from my daughter's home. He was also supportive of alternative therapies, such as massage and acupuncture.

The next morning I called him from my daughter's, pleading for an appointment, and he got me in late that afternoon. I was moving into critical mass and was starting to lose grasp of reality, accompanied with fatigue and a physical sense of death. I packed up my personal belongings and left Tassa and her boyfriend an "in-the-event-of-death" to-do list. I'm sure they sensed my state because I was beyond screening my reality from anyone.

I walked into Dr. David's office and sat on his couch. He asked briefly what was going on and I told him. He checked my muscle strength and said he felt there was nothing wrong with me physically in an organic sense, but said I was filled with intensity. Well, if he felt like me, he would be a little intense, too. After all, I was dying.

He said he was going to write me a perscription and I should take it and come back the next day, because I was just too intense to deal with today. I left and followed his instructions. The perscription was for Xanax, which I took immediately; I took another tablet several hours later.

My peripheral energy field relaxed a bit, as I became softly separated from both current and altered realities. *I will have to wait 'til tomorrow,* I thought, *before the doctor admits me to the hospital.*

With plodding energy, I made it through to the next day with my customary three to four hours of sleep. I arrived at Dr. David's office a bit more relaxed around the periphery, though heavily distraught at the core level.

This time he looked at me and surmised that I had been on a very long trajectory heading toward this moment. I told him that I no longer felt safe and felt as if I needed to go somewhere. He looked at me and said there was no place to go. There was no place between the hospital and home.

I asked how that could be; all I wanted was a place to go and feel safe. I learned at that moment that our society has a great hole in its service system, one that is surely going to grow. As a result, I asked if he could admit me to the hospital. He said, "No."

He stated that he wasn't sure that the hospital was the answer for me. He said that the emergency room was a crap-shoot and that, once in, they more than likely would put me on some heavy medication and send me home.

Deeply discouraged, I assessed my path as marginal, pointed directly into the heart of Mordor. He told me some very important things, such as he didn't know where I was going or how I had gotten here, but that I had been on my way for a long time.

He said if I were to write down my story, I might discover a clue as to what was transpiring. I left that day feeling like I had a thread in my hand that was connected to a tapestry of darkness. The following days at my daughter's consisted of my trying to do some phone work for my business and wandering occasionally out of my back bedroom into the backyard and sometimes down the block. The city was like a cage to me and I felt like an animal from another planet.

The medication — Lexipro, Clonazepam, and Xanax — was only medicating the semblence of what I sensed as my former reality. My entrapment in another dimension or reality was starting to calcify and disallow my movement back and forth.

I remember one afternoon when I was forced into the fetal position in the grass in my daughter's backyard. I could not emerge from the plane of my entrapment. It was like being dead and still breathing, in that the void of separation had a definitive eternity associated with it. The dark fear of this condition is ineffable, at best, and leaves one with ideas of suicide. Somehow I made it through that afternoon into the evening, realizing I could not go on like that in this space and time.

The next day, I called a psychiatrist friend, who told me to go to the emergency room but be sure to tell them that I couldn't take care of myself and that I was suicidal. She said the University of Washington was perhaps the best hospital choice. I also called Dr. David, who said to go for it, so I did.

I got all of my bank information and important papers together for my daughter and asked her boyfriend to drive me to the emergency room, wondering what on this planet would become of me. My daughter's boyfriend, by the way, was a gamer and took all of this in great stride.

We pulled up to the hospital and I got out and walked into the emergency room, ready for safe space and help. The intake that day was perfect; there was only one other person in the waiting room. I gave the reception nurse my name and he gave me a bracelet and told me to have a seat.

The thoughts that ran through my head were many, and a humorous one always found its way to the surface, because I would never have imagined my current plight. I was supposed to be training at the Healing Light Body School as opposed to jumping into a large crevasse completely alone.

They soon called my name and I went into the ER through the swinging doors, where they set upon me with body function equipment. The nurse asked why I was there and I said I thought I was dying and could no longer function in the world out there. She then asked if I was on any medication and if I felt like I could do harm to myself. I told her the medication I was on and said, yes, I could do harm to myself.

After the first cursory level of body testing, I was put in a side room off of the main corridor. I called my office and my parents and told them I was going into the hospital. My parents and business partner were supportive of whatever I needed.

Next, another nurse came in to check some other body functions while a doctor was summoned. I was then hooked up for an electrocardiogram, which revealed I was in tremendous shape (with body functions of a thirty-year-old). Again, I truly felt at this time that I needed to see an endocrinologist who would right the world with my diagnosis of a grave illness. No matter how I tried, I could never get one to appear.

The doctor came in and said all of my tests looked good and asked again what was going on. I listed my portfolio of causative circumstances: loss of children, daughter who just had a biopsy, father with cancer, best friend with stroke, homeless, dying of some unknown disease and psychosis. He seemed to grasp the situation and said he would get a caseworker.

A social worker showed up shortly and was very empathetic to my cause. She said she would find a bed for me in "7 North" (the psychiatric ward). I was very ready to experience whatever was so sanctioned.

The social worker walked me to the elevator and we exited at the seventh floor and walked to the locked entrance of 7 North. A buzzer unlocked the door and we entered; I was greeted by a kind woman and asked to check in at the front desk.

After some basic questions and answers, I was taken to a conference room where all of my belongings were checked. I called my daughter and asked her to bring my clothes (which I packed for the occasion) and my living will (which was prepared for a hospital visit). I got done checking in what little I had with me, and my daughter came to the locked door with her boyfriend, my son and his girlfriend. We hugged in a field of fear and humor. There I was, in a locked wing of the hospital, receiving clothes from my children. It was a good moment to try to assure them I would be fine, based on the circumstances.

All medication that I had with me was taken away. The one thing that remained was my hunger. They ordered me some soup and a sandwich, which was perfect.

I was shown to my room and introduced to my roommate, John. John had some anxiety surrounding his girlfriend and the loss of their relationship. He had a clear light and was one of the leaders of the 7 North tribe. The tribe was always evolving, pending the inflow and outflow of members. Some where longer-term members, who witnessed the changing of the guard over periods of time.

John slept in the bed next to the window and my bed was close to the door, with a pull divider separating the two and dividing the isle between us. We shared a bathroom with the room next to us. The door could be locked if someone from the other side occupied it. There were a series of nice shower stalls along the hall and all we had to do was ask for someone (a nurse or attendant) to unlock one.

The first evening I was given some Ambien (5 mg) and it did not work. After that, they adjusted the dose up to 10 mg, along with Clonazapin, and that did the trick. It was the first night I had slept five to seven hours in over six months.

I took a shower early every morning after some yoga and sit-ups. I was ususally the first or second person up on the floor at around 6 A.M. After my shower, I would have some decaf coffee and check my email messages. I liked it there.

I was introduced to the other participants on my second day, at our obligatory morning meeting. The structure was a blessing to me and was something to look forward to.

Every morning and afternoon we would have a community meeting and discuss the schedule for the rest of the shift, regarding nurse assignments and classes. The classes were geared to reorientation and skill development with regard to living in the world. People were assigned different classes in accordance with their condition. We had classes in which we played board games and classes for tai chi. Videos were always available. The meals were human in that we could pick from a vegetarian menu and order Garden Burgers. They did not have organic vegetables, but that day is coming.

The program in general seemed right up my alley. I had a safe place with an exceptional nursing staff and good-hearted medical doctors. During my first full day, I was introduced to my medical team, Team Purple, which consisted of several doctors, a few counselors and some doctor trainees.

When I was called in for my first spotlight session, I was asked what was going on. I felt like Arlo Guthrie doing a new version of "Alice's Resturant." After I was done reciting my causative conditions, the doctor asked me about suicidal thoughts and I said I had them. He asked me if I felt like hurting myself now and I said I did not. Lastly, I said, "I really need your help." He let me know he heard me and would, in fact, help me. His assessment was that I would be out of there in five days.

Hmm, I thought, *it feels like it is going to take longer than five days but I will take that as a good sign.*

Leaving the meeting, I asked again if I could see an endocrinologist. The doctor said he would see after my blood work results came back. I left feeling like the Purple Team could help me in some way, especially after my blood test came back, indicating that I was the picture of health, with no red flags pertaining to endocrinological issues. My quest for the omniscient and ever illusive endrocrinologist continued.

☆ ☆ ☆

Each day brought with it a varied dimension of perception as my medication was increased. After several days, I was given Level 3 status, allowing me to go outside two times a day, morning and evening, unsupervised. I used the mornings to go for a light run and sometimes found someone to throw the frisbee with in the afternoon. We always had an evening walk at 7 P.M. with everyone who could go out. We would find a place the smokers could enjoy, usually down by the water.

Days passed as different tribe members left to go back into the world; others were admitted in their place. When I left, only two original people out of fifteen were still there and they were planning to leave the day after. There were several long-care members who had been there for months, but the goal from the hospital's perspective was to get us out in five to seven days, pending our insurance.

Most who are dealt back into the world are not yet ready to resume normalcy. When my time came, I was better but still not capable of resuming my life as I had known it.

* * *

One of the most interesting events of my stay was the day I was asked if I would allow an interview in front of a class of practicing psychiatrists. I said yes and was escorted down to a teeming classroom full of fifteen to twenty student psychiatrists and a professor.

I sat in a chair at the front of the class with the professor next to me. He started the questioning: How did you get here? How do you feel? And so on.

As I had told the Purple Team, I said I was straddling realities along with a chronic hormone imbalance due to something that would never show up on a test. I mentioned again that I really wanted to see an endocrinologist. I took several questions from the students and that was that. The professor sent me off with his best regards and I was escorted back up to 7 North.

I was neutral about the experience and still am, assuming I was being quantified as a classic case of something. The hospital diagnosed me as a depressive type with some acute anxiety in the mix. I was depressed, no doubt, and anxious, but not for the reasons they surmised.

The bright spot of the care was the nursing staff, both male and female. The women in general had a shamanistic element that was comforting; one of them gave me an article about a shamanic practitioner in Hawaii. They did not come out and say anything specific about my condition but were embrasive of a larger context. This was comforting, though I did not know why.

The male nurses were also wonderful and supportive in a more linear and accepting way. It was a place I could have stayed another week, specifically because I had no real home to go back to. I still felt very weak and disoriented but was given my walking papers seven days out. The team did provide a thoughtful exit strategy by setting up counseling and psychiatric contacts for immediate assistance and reintegration. At $1,200 plus a day, it was a spendy stay, even with good insurance.

✲ ✲ ✲

The day before I was to be released, I made the necessary phone calls to my daughter and friends, deciding upon a pathway. Where was I going to go, since I was unable to work and had no money?

I decided to go back to my daughter's and stay the night then pack up and go back to my vacant home on Whidbey and figure it out. I had come upon one option for housing but the energy of the "landlord" was a bit militaristic and I needed something soft like butter, so I let that option go and waited for something to appear.

I stayed in the empty Whidbey house that was for sale and started to crumble at the core. This was early August and I found a wonderful spot to move but not until mid-September, so I had to live in a empty environment alone for many weeks. This is the period that ripped and clawed at my life force and my sense of being. I became acutely aware of my dying on all levels, yet I had to keep going alone.

I was undergoing a spiritual crisis in that it encompassed a dizzying array of conditions that I now understand as process points. At the time, however, I was utterly alone in the quandary of my insanity and physical debilitation. I could hardly function, though I kept up a façade for my business phone calls and my children, both of which were relying upon my continuance.

After many such calls, I would go into my empty living room in an altered daze and sit in a corner, feeling completely unsafe with nowhere to go for help. I started to experience intense energy currents that would run throughout my body, often forcing me to the floor and into a fetal position. I went through most all of these experiences completely alone, without human contact. I longed to the depth of being for a safe place in which to go through this stage of the ordeal, but could not find one.

It was then that an old friend who was wise about the process resurfaced, and was of magical support. She became openly available and supportive of what I needed. She also directed me to the Spiritual Emergence Network, where I located two transpersonal psychologists who, by divine circumstance, lived on Whidbey Island. They were the only two transpersonal psychologists practicing the facilitation of spiritual emergence in the state of Washington. A phone call to them set in motion the apexual stage of my process journey.

My divisional set of worlds continued, except that now, for the first time in over two years, I had a context upon which to nest the experience. It did little to assuage the daunting intensities, but did — along with the promise of Vedic astrology — offer me a potential way out.

The keystone book of this stage was *Healing through the Dark Emotions: The Wisdom of Grief, Fear and Despair,* by Miriam Greenspan. It is in my opinion one of the major works on transformation. I religiously kept it by my side in the ensuing months of transpersonal work.

I was still in my empty home, waiting for my newly located rental cottage to be completed. I began working with a transpersonal psychologist and began to refine my life's vision in broad sweeps.

Chapter V: The Path, Shunya

✧ ✧ ✧

Death, the Void, fear and eternities of darkness all stalked me through the following months.

In the latter part of August, I was wakened on a regular basis at 4 or 5 A.M. by electric energy running throughout my body. I would most often be forced out of my bed to the floor, where I would hang on to the side of the bed and writhe. I would always call my therapist, sometimes in the wee hours, and, if she wasn't available, would derive comfort from just listening to the voice message. My other dear friend, who was present for me, would also field my often frantic phone calls and reassure me of my permanence on the planet.

The days passed and I shouldered my aloneness as best I could. I was continually in search of safe space, since my solitary confinement and condition felt like a prescription for death, natural or induced. To be in what felt like a deteriorating space, locked out of my former reality with nowhere to go, was like a living death.

It was at this juncture that I started journeying, with the assistance of my therapist. It provided me with a starscape of information and a pathway through Mirkwood. The most important first step was to learn that I was okay and was going to be okay. The process, not for everyone, was a natural one for me. A higher part of myself realized the implicit truth. I realized begrudingly at first that, yes, I had to go through this completely and, yes, it was okay to go through this. I finally gave myself permission and I went.

The following is a list of concepts that came to me while I was journeying through the last stages of my process. It is a list that summarizes and highlights my experience.

Trust

Trust is one of the most powerful concepts to embrace. For me, Trust was the last crystal in the medicine bag, in that I had exhausted all else. When you feel like you are dying and no one can explain it empirically, you are given last rites to the task of Trust. When your tactile reference points are stripped away from you and Spirit is the most tangible truth around you, Trust takes form. It grows from Spirit down, vibrationally arriving as a connective link to an ineffable energy that intones within your acceptance and spiritual confidence toward an outcome sanctioned by love.

I trusted when I had nothing else and often struggled to find just a thread of Trust amidst my quest for survival. When I accepted my condition, Trust found me.

Love and Compassion

In the evolution of the process, one is opened to the simpler denominators of existence. Love and compassion are primary energy links to all life and existence. As I moved through the years of this process, love and compassion grew into a primacy of energy, an energy that became an essential first lens of observation.

Meditation and shamanic journeying help in solidifying these forces in one's daily life. Once touched by the simplicity of this feeling energy, the scar becomes eternal.

Self-Love and Unconditonal Love

Acceptance of self amidst the quandary of bodily self-defeat is of primacy and becomes clear often after an exhaustive bout with self-doubt and self-abnegation. Self-love evolves and did evolve for me as a baseline of acceptance.

Not unlike the pathway of Elizabeth Kubler Ross's work, *Death and Dying,* in which there are a series of understandings on the way to acceptance, spiritual crisis elicits an individual process. Self-love becomes a baseline of orientation that evolves into a broader scope of unconditional love and, hence, the acceptance of not only self, but all life around you. One becomes peaceful and at peace with the reality within and around oneself as a knowing of impermanence, amidst permanence, grows to maturation. All becomes acceptable within the context of self-love and unconditional love for all life.

Spirit World

Soon, in the process, one often becomes accustomed to more refined layers of reality. As the grosser levels of reality prove to be vaporous and slippery to the soul, the spiritual world emerges as a more accessible focal point for comraderie and connection. There is, it seems, a natural gravitation to the spiritual world as one is cast into the maelstrom of spiritual crisis. As all the tie ropes are ripped from the dock of normalcy, one realizes the all-inclusive sea of the spiritual domain, with its allure of eternal permanence amidst the temporal island of physical reality.

In many respects, the spiritual world becomes a new home for the crisis participant, affording connective comfort in a way far transcending comfort derived from the physical world. This domain often characterizes spiritual crisis, as one's attunement shifts to inclusion of a multidimensional reality. Once seen and experienced, it is difficult to rebuff, deny, and disengage from.

Fear

As though it were etched into all the subtle bodies of the crisis participants, fear surfaces time and time again, attempting to claim hegemony over all of one's emotions. In its relentless pursuit for emotional dominance, fear rolls in waves, often with tsunami force, submerging the crisis participant in a black, watery grave of insurmountable terror and confusion. It was beyond any fear I had experienced up to this point in my life. Days upon weeks of Void sparkled with gleamings of my former reality, with no means of rejoinder. I reached out to, but was unable to touch, the fabric of my former life or any life void of acute anxiety, depression, altered states, physical trauma, and death.

Day after day of crawling on the floor with bouts of energy emission and shaking, behind a façade of normalcy, redefined within me what fear felt like, how it tasted and smelled. I told myself that if I made it out of this crisis alive, I would do whatever I could to help lessen the anguish and pain of others in this process because I would never want another being to feel the fear that I felt. It is a theme common with crisis participation and post-crisis commitment.

Death

The ultimate journey of death beckons the crisis participant with an all-expenses-paid, first-class seating adventure. Death lives continuously just around the corner in our normal reality and, during the process, moves into the passenger seat with direct eye contact. One is forced into the acceptance of death, like it or not. The key is how one embraces this stern reality.

Often, during my process, I entertained the idea of suicide, feeling that if I had to continue in the space I was in, I would prefer to take my chances rolling the dice on the infinity of the bardo plane. I refrained, though there were times I came very close to driving off the road, hoping it would be perceived as an accident. Death can move from an abstract position to a tenable option then the reality of your present state and condition.

The death process evolves over time into a multilayered understanding of not only physical death, but the death of one's parts and layers. Elements of one's being no longer serve the soul's journey and must be released. We are all dying on a day-to-day basis, physically, emotionally, and spiritually shedding parts that are no longer needed. This happens subtly and, when experienced in crisis, blatantly.

Death happens between lives as life happens between deaths. Our choice is to embrace with love the continuum, or not. The spiritual crisis tends to illuminate the continuum.

Timeless Entrapment

Being caught in the Void with no way out is often associated with spiritual emergence. It is like being locked in a transparent room from which you observe your former reality and are unable to interact with or access its frequency or vibrational pattern.

I often felt like I was dead and yet could see and percieve my former vibrational plane, unable to recalibrate or access it. These stints in the transparent room would happen with regularity leaving, me adrift and groundless.

For weeks upon weeks, I would shudder at having to go out into "that world" and function. I saw people happy and going about their absolutely normal existence, and saw how I could not. I did not honestly think it would ever change. Why should it? I had no feedback, until the end, that it would. I thought that I would have to live the rest of my life in some institution — and I had made peace with that thought, knowing I had no other tangible option.

Moving into the present, along with surrendering, allowed me an opening to crawl through. As I gained perspective and was gifted with a spiritual crisis diagnosis, I began to gain confidence as to my emergence out of the timeless Void.

Merging Worlds

Love is an upliftment of the vibrational frequency level of "normal reality." "As above, so below" becomes a clear axiom for integrational observation and acceptance of reality. Connectivity is heightened, and joy becomes a corollary of rightful attentive action. Meditation now extends from a point of stillness to conscious observation of the world. The same lens is in use, though at a variant degree of magnification with the sitting, stillness, breath-oriented quietude state. Linkage is sustained.

Freedom, joy, and love are affirmations of this connection with source — not objectives, but results. It allows and accepts this state as is, amidst the almost gravitational pull of distraction. Discernment and witnessing allow (and allow one to choose) attention toward events supportive to connection and compassion, as well as toward events of a disconnective nature, so that all events become connective.

Heat

Another element inherent to my process was flushing and body heat, experienced almost to the hour on a daily basis (usually in the afternoon). This was perceived by the medical trust as an anomaly associated with illness. I was diagnosed with everything from an aberrant strand of malaria to mercury poisoning and adrenal faliure.

The heat, it turned out, was a cleansing element that preceded the electric energy streams that had their way with my body. Not one medical professional grasped the intrinsic value of this heat and almost all of the medical practitioners, both allopathic and alternative, wanted to stop it cold.

These components of the process were considered normal in antiquity, whereas, in current global medicine, they are viewed as pathological. Only near the end of my experience was I informed by my transpersonal psychologist that the heat was often customary in such a process.

Insomnia

Sleep was one of the first functions that started to herald my bodily changes. Eight to twelve months before the apex, my sleep started to become altered and minimized. I took every natural sleep aid available, finally ending with Sleepez, a heavy hitter from Canada.

Struggling often to get more than four hours of moderate, low-REM sleep, my body weakened. I awoke in the wee hours of the morning with night sweats for many months.

I feel that sleep is obviously vital and must be given high priority thoughout the process. In my instance, I was viewed as an entity with multifactorial symptoms and not an entity moving through a process holistically: Kali Yuga(The Iron Age) on the way to Dwapara Yuga(Bronze Age).

Isolation

This concept is fascinating in that it is one of the most frightening experiences and, at the same time, one of the most essential. I was alone most of the time through the apex of my experience and feel that it was a vital and essential component to passing through the experience. I could not have processed to the necessary extent had I been in a conventional social environment preceding my experience.

I feel that the axiom of not being able to solve a dilemma on the same plane of its conception is applicable to isolation. You do have to go it alone, without your partner or family, for a period of time in order to fully acclimate to a new way of being. I see many in prolonged experiences not willing to forego their accustomed lifestyle and relationship patterning. This is a moot point and one that will, I am sure, incur scorn from many.

I was on another level experiencing Sade Sati, which is about loss on many levels, so my condition was sanctioned and I had loss without choice. In the final analysis, I do believe it was crucial to the expedience of the process.

Physical Illness

Physical illness and its cause is a dissertation unto itself. My case involved a protracted series of symptoms, which were viewed from an allopathic, orthomolecular, naturopathic, Chinese, and ayurvedic perspective. I had a potpourri of symptoms with a multifactoral diagnosis that streched over two years.

Leading the parade was the ever-popular chronic fatigue, the catch-all for "I really don't know what it is," then on to mercury poisoning, mold toxicity, amalgam poisoning, Lyme disease, etc. I literally became a depository for hundreds of natural supplements.

The practitioners I saw were all at the top of their game, and all looked at it from their unique perspectives and treated it with their legally dealt supplements. I look back, smiling, at the ordeal I experienced in the hands of what many describe as the leading alternative doctors in their respective fields.

The Chinese perspective was positive and supportive, but the most profound was the ayurvedic, as administered by a true ayurvedic doctor. The reality was that my illness stemmed from a spiritual and mental energetic, a so-called Vatta imbalance, and was not simply an autonomous somatically-generated phenomenon (and I believe all illness is so governed). I was in the medical white waters for over two years before anyone suggested a psychiatrist or psychologist.

Interestingly, I was around a medical community that had been self-ordained as holistic. They understood positive attitudes and the spiritual, but had no protocol for inclusion as a diagnosis/prognosis. I remember my ayurvedic doctor responding to my query as to how he would address my myriad of symptoms; he looked at me and said, "I am not concerned about the soldiers. I am addressing the general." Up to that point, all of the practitioners I had seen (except for the Chinese physician) had been focused on making the soldiers go away via truckloads of mega-priced supplements, available more often than not at their in-office pharmacy.

The ayurvedic science, based on the Tridosha system of balancing Vatta, Kapha, and Pitta, makes basic sense and is founded on what I believe is over 10,000 years of experience. It is about the generals, balance, and cleansing, which, if used in conjunction with a good transpersonal therapist, can be an expansive solution. Illness can be a psychosomatic phenomenon and should be treated accordingly.

Prayer (Help, Appreciation, Surrender)

Prayer is a clear, individual process and is a key component to regaining and maintaining health. It is a conscious invitation for connection with the divine and subsequent connection with our eternal nature.

Opening to our brethren and sistern of the subtle worlds affords us communion with healing and balancing energies, only now being hypothesized via quantum physics and mechanics. Prayer works and becomes viable, as the veil of separation thins concurrently with our accelerated rate of planetary evolution and multidimensional access.

The prayer continuum that has proved helpful for me is tripartite in essence: first, seeking help and guidance as to my path and condition; secondly, appreciation and gratitude for all that I have been graced with; and lastly, surrendering to "thy will be done" with love and compassion.

Grounding

The process of grounding is a tool and ally in the emergency/emergence process. The energy that is released and processed during the experience needs to be facilitated and grounded. Mother Earth beckons to receive your energy on the out-breath and purifies the energy to be returned on the inbreath.

Grounding was one of the most stabilizing practices I used and it balanced an often-frenetic energy pattern. Many people I have talked to who have had energy imbalances also found profound relief from a grounding practice. It is a lifesaving tool for emergency crisis management.

Breath

Breath is perhaps the number-one ally in crisis management. Watching your breath and fully bringing your existence into the Now is often the only tool we have at our disposal.

Breath allows attention to frame the immediate moment and allows for a break in the mental continuum of an eternal crisis scenario. Attentive breathing can link Now moments into positive interludes, as one rushes down the rapids of fear and disorientation. Breath is also a calming practice and, most importantly, evokes your divine connection with Spirit.

Coping with the Darkness

The path of the crisis more often than not brings one into proximity of, then squarely into, the energy of the Darkness. ***This must be clearly felt and understood!***

Our culture has created an anti-Darkness socialization system in which the Darkness is cast as an evil, negative force that is to be turned away from and avoided at all costs. I and others, including Mariam Greenspan, feel that the Darkness is our greatest teacher and one that we must learn to embrace. Death, loss, fear, grief, and despair are all great teachers that we must learn to dance with.

In my experience, a crisis amplifies and illuminates the Darkness and directs us to its gift as an ally. The Darkness is immense and clearly subject to the soul's individuation. No two souls are going to experience the same color of Darkness, but both will need to access the same unifying quality of Light as it illumines the wisdom and elicits the teachings from the dark crystal's deep beauty. The Darkness must then be enjoined and mixed into the internal cauldron of processing, freeing its essences to blend with the aromatic scents of Light.

"You Create Your Reality" School

This is an interesting angle of energetics in that it corroborates an axiom and, at the same time, causes consternation on behalf of someone in crisis. Many people that I know who are advocates for creating your reality have, or have had, a safe financial base. I have unfortunately seen this financial advantage over used as justification for reality creating talent.This does not alter the truth of being positive or advocating any number of positivistic schools of thought, from Abraham Hicks, Hendrix, Dyer, etc.

Many, however, minimize the actual experience of going through a necessary and challenging stage of growth, instead casting the experience as a simple create your reality Faux pas .Yes, we can create our health and reality within the context of our Karma and divine pathway. However, I believe we cannot shun the often necessary pathway of transformation as it envelopes us and casts us into an emotional and physical Darkness.

Without having achieved a fully enlightened status, some of us are destined to experience change in the old-fashioned way, by groveling in the mire of insanity and illness in order to create our reality. It is important to note that the process is temporary and that there is a timeframe to the emergence. Once traction is achieved, it is vital to optimize your thoughts and actions toward health and the unification and sanctity of all life. To this end may your reality be created.

Now

From Eckart Tolle, Ram Dass, and Osho to all the saints and saviors, the concept of Now is the benchmark of attentive existence and the one doorway to eternity. It is, for the experiencer, a mantra of existence amidst mind-flooding torrents of eternal damnation and infinitudes of irreconcilable realities.

The true power of Now lies amidst the silent, relaxed acceptance of the moment, filled with gratitude and prayer. The Trust that accompanies this acceptance is bolstered by the flowering of one moment into the next, corroborating one's existence and breath.

Now serves as a link to an eternity of moments that change and eventually allow for freedom from the servitude and chains of seemingly inescapable Darkness and despair. Now is the door into the chapel of salvation.

Dharma

One's Dharma, or purpose, is often revealed as a corollary to the emergence experience. A crisis often serves as a catalyst for some degree of definitive change, the depth of which can only be surmised by the individual.

One's purpose in a lifetime is often relegated to the backburner of priorities and stews, sending wafts of unfulfilled contracts through fields and, eventually, the infrastructure, as it is somatized within the physical system.

Most medical practitioners don't ask, within the context of physical disease and illness, if you feel connected to actualizing your Dharma in this lifetime, but they should. It is clear that bringing one's Dharma into conscious realization is vital to health and happiness, and non-recognition creates illness and disease.

The emergence crisis phenomenon is as much about individuals and planets awakening to purpose as it is anything else. For those going through a crisis, it is important that the concept of Dharma be offered as an emergent realization that allows, in degrees, context for one's changing sense of being. Actualization of one's Dharma can be the gold ring at the end of the experiencer's journey.

Patience

The ultimate virtue, especially when one is in crisis, patience is a difficult sell to one being bandied about within the standard medical model, which is usually bent on symptomatic relief.

Patience as a concept became acceptable only when I left the allopathic/naturapathic/alternative model and embraced the ayurvedic/spiritual/transpersonal model, which accounted for a set duration for the crisis experience.

Without proper guidance from experienced practitioners, one can easily drift into the mindset of eternal suffering. As my experience proved, there is a severe disconnect between the reality of subtle body trauma and the resultant physical body illness.

I believe that a staggering number of people are harmed by standard and "alternative" medical systems. Patience comes with a knowing of duration and due process, and no other way.

Medical

The medical pathway I followed was not only costly but emotionally exhausting. Untold millions, I feel, are locked into a stalled process of emergence primarily due to the medical community on the planet today. Their effort to thwart and curtail a natural process is evidenced by the millions of people on antidepressants and marginally understood drugs. I believe chronic fatigue is a process illness, as are most adrenal-associated illnesses.

The majority of practitioners — as my ayurvedic doctor said — are out to defeat the soldiers and perhaps get lucky and win a battle, whereas the real work is in defeating the general and winning the war. This can only be accomplished by embracing a holistic, inclusive approach, not unlike ayurveda, with supplemental transpersonal psychology and energy work.

The alternative medical establishment, for the most part, is as unbalanced in its approach as the allopathic, and both are making a lot of money by keeping people in a static medical position.

Allopathic

There are, of course, caring and exceptional doctors in the world; however, in general, you want to bypass this pathway if you feel you are in a spiritual crisis. I was fortunate to have a creative psychiatrist who was a meditator and knew I had to go through whatever it was I was going through. Most, however, pride themselves in talk therapy and sedation via Prosac, Lexapro, etc.

When it comes to mechanical fixes, allopathic medicine has its pluses, but needs to be blended with spiritual energetic practices, i.e., transpersonal therapy, shamanic healing, etc., if it hopes to have efficacy for an evolutionary culture.

Orthomolecular

This approach has its place, as do all healing modalities per the evolution of the patient. Treating imbalances with pills is good to a point, and this is the crux of orthomolecular medicine, which is basically a "hit 'em where they ain't" approach in that natural supplements and drips can restore an imbalance. Linus Pauling and vitamin C mega-approaches are great if you believe in them, but are probably not so effective if you don't.

Ayurveda

Balancing the primacy of the Tridosha system (Vatta, Kapha, Pitta) implicitly makes the most sense to me. Inherent to this system is spiritual imbalance and causative planetary imbalance. Finding a bonafide vs. weekend-certified practitioner is important. A true practitioner is one who has spent a lifetime in service and practice, because 10,000 years of data is a lot to absorb.

Acupuncture

Balancing the body through 'energy meridian activation' is a tremendous supplement to cleansing work and is potent as an energy balancing system. Finding a big-picture practitioner is again the key. I was blessed in finding one who also practiced energy work and I would certainly suggest the combination, if possible.

Jin Shin Jitsu

This practice was highly effective in balancing my energy and came at a divine time. I was fortunate to experience this practice in conjunction with the Kaya Kalpa, and it kept me tethered to the planet.

There were days I could hardly walk into the treatments and become revitalized to the degree that I could easily walk out. Balancing your treatments per your constitution and temperament is an important, intuitive process that each person must enact. Energy work must accompany whichever healing practice is adopted.

Energy Work

The essential nature of all life is energy, and clearly it is so with human beings. As our subtle bodies become activated with information and energy from light realms, there is a natural decompression and transfer of energy to the physical body. This transfer is often in concert with the recodifing of the genetic celluar system, and requires adaptation on behalf of the physical body.

Untold numbers of illnesses are directly associated with this adaptational process and need skilled midwifery in regard to holding sacred space and working with the body to facilitate process, not stop it. Energy work is the medicine of the present/future.

Chiropractic

Having an enlightened chiropractor is certainly an advantage. Chiropractic treatment is a great healing service, specifically with structural physical imbalances. It is a blessing to be connected to a wise one. I would recommend it as one of the positive healing modalities.

Massage

Massage is magical when received from an attentive practitioner who is clear on the ways of giving. Human touch can easily be divine when given by a clear channel. As one goes through process, one of the greatest gifts is to have access to clear light massage. As your body adapts to the energy and information from subtle fields, it is a grace to have someone facilitate the transfer by touch.

Most people in crisis are intuitively guided to the right massage practitioner for them, or the right one somehow appears. There are many styles of massage for the many types of people and souls that would benefit from them. It is a keystone of healing for the crisis-emergent soul.

Counseling

"Buyer, beware" is extremely applicable for counselors in general. If they are not an experiencer, I would keep moving until you find one who has been though an emergence experience. Most counselors are kind and, of course, helpful to a point. But when it comes down to knowing how to guide one through a spiritual crisis, most, unfortunately, do not have the experience or training. Hence, I recommend transpersonal counseling.

Transpersonal Counseling

I was fortunate to find transpersonal counselors when I did, via the Spiritual Emergence Network. There is a branch in the United States and in Canada. The transpersonal counselor is primarily an offshoot of the work done on spiritual crisis by Dr. Stanislav Grof, in that most practitioners have studied his work extensively. As the transpersonal work evolves, I suspect it will take on more shamanic attributes. I was helped immensely by the process of journeying, which is often associated with shamanic work.

The evolution of the planet and the enlivening of the noosphere demand an evolved psychology system, and transpersonal psychology seems to be on track with that stream of evolution. I rate it highly for someone in spiritual and/or emergency crisis.

Meditation

The process of 'dropping the mind' is consistent with all practices involving unity. It is in the silence that all is heard. Setting aside time to be silent and connected to the source through breath is a vital link in establising a quality connection with Spirit and the eternity of Now.

Meditation can represent the stepping stones as you wade down the river of process and crisis until you reach the invitational sea of unification and are beckoned to jump in. All aspects of process uniquely reflect each soul's journey and requirements. Some may need to meditate more and others less. Each of us must find our own balancing Mandala/Yantra of energetic patterning.

Unity

Unification becomes the means, as opposed to the objective, when one is in process. One is often forced to redefine relationships to all life during a crisis experience and unity is made manifest through observation and one's proximity to the source.

Connectivity to the source becomes actualized through a series of reducive experiences, after which all that is left is Spirit. The experiencer has been stripped of all extraneous connection and, through silence and total alone-ness, finds the unity of all things. It is usually afterward that the experiencer finds a heightened degree of peace along their respective pathway, and sometimes not a moment too soon.

Acceptance often hides in Trust's shadow as one is relegated to a one-on-one experience with unity. The experiencer must trust the safety of the inclusionary step into unity, whereby the differentiation of individuation gives way to a shared energy with all existence and time.

Astrology Jyotish

This Science of Light is a system that predates most astrological systems and is a lifetime pursuit, if studied properly. My experience with Jyotish stems from my own practice of it as a science. The benefit to a soul in crisis is clear in that often, and with a high degree of accuracy, a timeframe can be applied to the experience based on planetary positioning. This is of immense benefit as one in crisis struggles with the eternity of certain conditions inherent to the process.

I was blessed by having an extremely gifted astrologer illuminate my pathway, heralding the day of my transformation and transfiguration. It is an important, if not vital, tool to access during one's process, and one that supports the reverence of change and transformation.

Psychic Interpretation

Throughout my journey, I was in contact with a spiritual psychic, one who glimpsed the future through a lens of love and compassion. The psychic field is full of spectrum-seers and I believe one attracts those who are in alignment with one's soul pathway. I was fortunate to have a heartful seer a phone call away who would provide an often needed cushioning to conditions that belied physical plane rational.

It is a field that will, I feel, gain more and more credibility as the fields surrounding the human body and planet become more discernible. We exist on many dimensions at once and are developing intuitive access to these dimensions at an exponential rate. A grounded, heartful psychic can lend tremendous support as one ventures into the darkened regions and peripheral terrain of existence.

Music

Classical music such as Debussy, Ravel, Wagner, Holst, Bach, etc., as well as world beat, chant, and etheric (stargate) music, all provide a positive energy during some of the sombering moments of crisis. A cup of tea and your favorite music can often soothe you like nothing else during such moments. Sounds of rushing water, birds singing, and wind chimes are also vital to the spirit and afford comfort in times of stress. Music is a beautiful component that should be explored in times of deep healing.

Your Story

Everyone should know their own story. It is a pivotal stage in any healing process and vital to one in crisis. When we clearly view the entirety of our life as a continuum, we can truly understand how we arrived in the present and what emotional terrain we have traversed to get here. Write down your story and you will be amazed at the cause and effect scenarios that emerge and clarify themselves before your very heart and eyes.

Compassion

Truly one of the most profound and adaptational concepts that emerges through the energy crisis process, compassion becomes a clarifying lens through which one sees oneself, the world, and humankind. It becomes necessary, since one is often left with a heightened sensitivity to dimensional energies. What are seen in many human beings as imbalances and often psychological tendencies become muted and understood in the context of universal compassion. It is a necessary and vital perspective in the light of heightened polarities amidst an evolutionary, planetary culture.

Surrender

There comes a point in an individual's process when one realizes the infinite potential for stasis vs. organic movement and completion. It is usually in the neighborhood of this juncture that Surrender surfaces as a viable option, after one has been locked in what can feel like a downward physiological spiral.

The acceptance of Surrender, releases the boundaries to 360 degrees of posssible outcome, ordained by divine providence. Thus, Surrender is the linchpin of complete acceptance. It comes with divine timing to allay the notion of disconnection, which is gracefully supplanted by the notion of unity and divine, loving causality.

Chapter VI: Process Facilities — The Vision, the Need

✲ ✲ ✲

Safety and Safe Space

Safety and safe space were my middle names throughout the latter stages of my process. I continually tried to find them. Daily, I struggled in my alone-ness and discomfort and longed for a simple bedroom setting where loving people were close at hand.

I knew I would have to complete the journey alone, but to have knowledgeable, loving companionship in the next room or down the hall would have made me smile. To have had someone bring me soup and tell me it was going to be okay became my mantra, as I crawled on the floor, growling and screaming for freedom.

Opening of the Heart

Perhaps one of the most profound experiences and turning points of my life occured after a fourteen-hour drive up and back to the middle of British Columbia, Canada, to attend a retreat of experiencers in a safe space.

The retreat was led by a self-advocated enlightened shaman. I should have known better, but I was in such a state of flux that I went with a flow that seemed to be marginally okay. I was told the space was safe and that it was a place I needed to be. I took off, packing all my basic necessities, and was prepared to vanish into the Canadian Rockies through the magic door of this "safe retreat led by an enlightened soul."

I arrived, exhausted and hungry, and was received with some degree of grace. I was not offered any food but was given tea and was told that "Ms. Y" would be down soon. I had inadvertently walked into a meditation room with my tea and was immediately chastised for entering with a beverage. I was so altered it did not matter, so I left to drink my tea in another room.

Soon we gathered (eleven total, five of whom were staff members). An announcement was made that the teacher was coming. By that time, I had started shaking due to the drive, my process, and where I was. One of staff wrapped me with a blanket and told me to sit against the wall as the teacher walked in. I accepted whatever was, because I had no other option.

What happened over the next three hours was enlightening to some, but to me it was an exercise in stamina. It was a great Spirituality 101 course, but not what I was led to believe would be taught. I was the only one shaking and I am sure the only one dangling by a single energtic thread.

After the event that evening, I went up to the teacher and said I was barely hanging on and felt I needed to scream and cry. She looked at me and said, "There are miles of forest behind the house that go on forever, if you need to go and scream."

Hmm, I thought, *this does not feel too good.* I said, "Thanks," pulled my staff friend aside, and said I would probably leave in the morning. She asked me to sleep on it.

I did, barely, and was up and ready to go at daybreak.

As I was leaving, I was confrontationally addressed by the teacher's lover, who told me I had no idea what I would be missing, that I did not have a clue as to what was going on there, and how could I be so uninsightful. I could only agree with him as I picked up my bags and walked out the door.

There I was, the day after a seven-hour drive, with very little sleep, having just been judged and juried, going out to my car on the road to nowhere, in the middle of British Columbia. I drove into downtown Kamploops and sought some directions at a café to get back to the highway.

At the café, I called my friend on Whidbey and my transpersonal therapist, who were both surprised by my abrupt exit from the safe space and my quest for Alice's rabbit hole, until I explained how unsafe it was. Both were encouraging and told me to keep them posted.

I decided to drive to Vancouver, where a friend had started a Spiritual Emergence Center. The only problem was that the center did not yet have a place to put someone in crisis, leaving me in the middle of British Columbia with no place to go to process.

I again called my transpersonal therapist, who saved the day by telling me to come back to Whidbey and stay at her house. Relieved, yet dissapointed as to my lack of traction to find Lothlorien, I went back to Whidbey and a welcoming from two helpful souls.

There, over the next several days, my heart opened. The opening followed a journey, whereby I leapt into molten lava and ascended with a spirit guide to visit my deceased son, Pir, who would be twenty-five this year, and my beloved dog, Cody, who was now Pir's dog.

Pir passed after a brief visit of one day in 1982. The visit illumined the unfinished business of my grief over and acknowledgement of Pir, and the undying love I have for my two living children, Tassa and Braelyn. My heart opened its eyes and became a new visual tool from which to see.

Letter (Dated 9/07/06)

We find ourselves amidst a flurry of subconscious to conscious need of an intermediary facility for people in the throes of a transformational spiritual process. This process has outdistanced the infrastructure (individual psychotherapy, psychiatric, and hospital psychiatric care) and now must focus on compassionate, facilitational, and understanding care. We are at the vanguard of a process facilitation revolution, grounded in spiritual evolution.

My process roots back twenty-seven years and has reached efflorescence over the last six months, whereby my former life and world has been completely taken away and a new restructured world has emerged. I have spent time at the University of Washington psychiatric ward as an inpatient and have undergone days and months of complete disorientation, accompanied by relentless energy flows throughout my body. I knew this time was coming and feared it for many years, yet also knew it was essential for me in order to complete my purpose in this lifetime. I held it off with all of my will until my son Braelyn, my last child, graduated from high school this past June.

My journeying and prayer has led me to my purpose: to be involved with other souls in the co-creation of Life/Transformational/Transition centers geared to individuals in Spiritual Crisis and Spiritual Emergence. A flagship facility is needed from which a documentary and book project will flow, highlighting the evolutionary need and exigencies for manifestation on a global basis. I see many levels in this unfolding. Primary is the grounding in love, compassion, and sacred-safe space.

I feel there will emerge an urban system geared to day-care emergency crisis treatment, staffed by a psychotherapist and an adjunct psychiatrist for medical consultation and medication on an as-needed basis. The intake procedure and determinism as to need is critical and pivotal to immediate protocol. Five to seven bedrooms would be optimal with, at a minimum, three room attendants. Providing an ambient energetic of safety, love, and compassion is key. One director per urban house would be needed to oversee financial and legal necessities.

A world liaison specialist would also be advisable to oversee the intake individual's worldly responsibilities, i.e., contacting significant others, holding mail, arranging for pet care, contacting workplace, etc. In short, interfacing on behalf of the person with her or his world is needed to minimize their stress on how to hold that world together.

For short stays of five to seven days, a reemergence facilitator would be on call to help orient and integrate worlds, so that functioning could be maintained. If a person requires more in-depth assistance then they would be moved to a pastoral ex-urban center.

This would be the hub of the operation, designed ideally on an energy location (Ley line confluence) using sacred geometric design systems. It would be holistic and staffed by a psychotherapist/psychiatrist, ayurvedic physician, body workers, shamanic practitioners, director, world liaison specialists, and a reemergence facilitator. Color and sound would be used as transformational tools along with aromatherapy. Access to water, set in a healing, natural environment, is vital.

The third possible level would be a group home where individuals could be moved after time in the treatment facility, for those who need more time to integrate worlds and internalize their process with the world around them. These homes could be established to exist on a cottage industry basis, fostering a spiritually based right-livelihood business, such as baking organic cookies or printing organic cotton and hemp T-shirts with positive messaging. In any event, a segue facility would be optimum for a certain percentage of individuals.

This is obviously just a sketch of possibilities with little grounded attention to the major component of funding. I do feel that a documentary and book project off of the flagship system will attract whatever is needed to proceed, perhaps the Gates Foundation, among others.

I am looking to work with people who share the spirit of this concept and am willing to move globally to be of service and be facilitational.

Chapter VII: Experiencers

✳ ✳ ✳

Brothering and Sistering

Once you have experienced a process of emergence, you now have an extended family of other experiencers, for it truly is like gaining an extensive lineage of brothers and sisters. The time is now for the brothering and sistering of the planet, and this is one modus of potent transcendant linkage via Pierre Teilhard de Chardin.

All the souls that I have met since my journey who have also journeyed the emergent path are instantly recognizable by word and/or deed. It is a common bonding, I suppose, like any co-shared death experience, but what emerges from the bonding is a shared, incessant desire to be of service to others in process and to facilitate the unity of life upon the planet. It is like sharing a universal implant geared to unificational planetary evolution.

The Spectrum of Process Experiencers

Energy medicine will continue to evolve as more and more individuals become self-realized within the context of their illness, disease, and psychological dilemma. The answer lies in the energetic realm or pre-somatic state.

Having been personally diagnosed with an array of illnesses by so-called cutting-edge, and not-so-cutting-edge, practitioners, I can say that the emergent edge of energy medicine is now at hand and will evolve exponentially. The fact that there are millions of people on psychotropic drugs, suffering with chronic "I don't know what it is-ness," shows that we are in a planetary crisis presaging a multidimensional transformation of all life.

Albeit Pierre Teilhard de Chardin's Ultra Hominisation, or the advent of fifth dimensional consciousness, heralds a new paradigm of reality. Steiner's fifth major cycle and fifth minor cycle timeframe is also represented at the present moment, capturing and codifying an expanded alternative time continuum (Chart A-B-C). The experiencers held captive in the following myriad conditions need relief and it will soon come to pass that they shall receive it.

The following conditions can and have been associated with transformative emergence and crisis:

Chronic fatigue syndrome

Lyme disease

Mercury posioning

Mold toxicity

Depression

Anxiety disorder

Post-traumatic stress disorder

Bipolar disorder

Kundalini awakening
Obsessive compulsive disorder
Fibromyalga
Rushes of energy
Psychic experiences
Mood swings
Past trauma resurfacing
Extreme sensitivity
Tremors/vibrations
Disassociation
Fear of the unknown and known
Hot flashes and bodily heat
Aches and pains
Extraterrestrial abduction
Clairaudience
Clairsentience
Clairvoyance
Etc.

Chapter VIII: Emergence/Emergency

✤ ✤ ✤

As the planet and its inhabitants emerge from a collective moment of 'what was' to 'what can be,' all elements are subjected to a vibrational, energetic adjustment. Such a change is perhaps predestined by innumerable factors, notwithstanding one's karmic, astrological, and self-realizational status; however, there are larger cycles that offer a conciliatory and compassionate perspective.

I. Steiner/Yugas

The theosophical chains and rounds, along with the anthroposophical septenary system (Chart A-B-C), illustrate a Westernized-esoteric perspective to ancient India's Yuga system. Sri Yukteswar's 24,000-year Yuga calendar is a great representative tool of the Indian system (Chart D).

We will briefly look at both of these, since they can account for the collective slothfulness in reference to the imminent dimensional shift in existence. Both sets of systems present a cyclic and/or spiralic movement to evolution, set amidst a continuum of pre-mist to post-mist dimensions.

The anthroposophical, 343-stage evolutionary system by Rudolph Steiner casts a long net in harnessing multidimensional time continuums beyond the periphery of commmon thought. Being a scientist of the spirit, Steiner posits the Major Septenary Cycle of Ancient Saturn, Sun, Moon, Earth, Venus, Jupiter, and Vulcan stretching back billions of years and emergent through many dimensions (Chart A). Each major cycle is comprised of seven minor cycles, each comprised of seven subminor cycles. We are currently in the fifth subminor cycle (Indian, Persian, Chaldean-Babalonian-Egyptian, Grecco-Latin), and the present is Earth's fifth minor cycle (Polarean, Hyperborean, Lemurian, Atlantian, present) [Charts B-C].

The 24,000-year Yuga system by Sri Yukteswar shows how, due to the revolution of the solar system around a dark companion star and our relativity to the Galactic Center, we are reflective of available consciousness.

When our solar system has a clear, unobstructed relationship with the Galactic Center, we are in a Satya Yuga or Golden Age. When the Galactic Center is blocked by the dark companion star, we experience a Kali Yuga or Iron Age (Chart D). We are, according to Sri Yukteswar, currently in the Dwapara Yuga (Bronze Age) and proceeding to the Treta Yuga (Silver Age).

This scenario amplifies the concept of available consciousness and affords compassion based on access to a limited supply of Galactic Center energy.

II. 2012

Our last foray into Satya Yuga was during the later years of the Atlantean culture, thirteen thousand to fourteen thousand years ago. Steiner's system and the Indian Yuga's both denote a quickening of the pulse of transformative evolution and allude to a less than apocryphal shift around the 2012 timeframe.

The Dwapara Yuga is nested in a larger Yuga cycle of 3,160,000,000,000 years, made up of 131,666,666 24,000-year minor Yugas, in which we are thought to be in a Kali or nadir phase.

Steiner, meanwhile, has periodic catastrophism built into his system, yet the next major catastrophic period should commence with the end of the seventh subculture of the fifth Major Earth Cycle, hundreds of thousands of years from now (Chart B).

Atlantis experienced episodic catastrophies over its existence, so we must conclude the likelihood is inherent in Steiner's system to account for periodic catastrophies. This would account for, or at least provide room for, a 2012 energetic shift.

So, with the dimensionality of time and consciousness, what potentially confronts us as we approach the much-heralded 2012, end of times, fourth into fifth dimension, etc., with a clear trend of emergence and emergency?

The Demarcation as seen from a planetary perspective:

- Hopi predict a twenty-five-year period of purification followed by the end of Fourth World and beginning of the Fifth.

- Mayans call it the "end days" or the end of time as we know it.

- Maoris say that as the veils dissolve, there will be a merging of the physical and spiritual worlds.

- The Zulu belief is that the whole world will be turned upside down.

- Hindus call it Kali Yuga (end time of man), the Coming of Kalki and critical mass of the Enlightened Ones.

- Incas call it the "Age of Meeting Ourselves Again."

- Aztecs call this the Time of the Sixth Sun, a time of transformation and creation of a new race.

- Dogon say that the spaceship of the visitors, the Nommo, will return in the form of a blue star.

- The Pueblo acknowledge it will be the emergence into the Fifth World.

- The ancient Cherokee calendar ends exactly at 2012, as does the Mayan calendar.

- The Tibetan Kalachakra teachings are prophesies left by Buddha predicting the Coming of the Golden Age.

- In Egypt, according to the Great Pyramid (stone calendar), the present time cycle ends in the year 2012 A.D.

And from a seer's perspective:

- "...a telepathic interplay, which will eventually annihilate time." (Alice Bailey)

- "...translation or dematerialization to another sphere of the Universe." (Teilhard de Chardin)

- "...a matter-antimatter implosion leaving a mutation of matter to photoniform. Our minds will unite like the fragments of a hologram." (Terence McKenna)

- "...as the Schumann resonance increases to 13 Hz, Gaia goes from Alpha to Beta frequency and wakes up. Increasing tryptamine and beta-carboline neuro-chemistry allows us a telepathic communion, as we become used to our light bodies in preparation for the magnetic pole reversal when there will be a mass out-of-body-experience." (Geoff Stray)

- "...evolutionary quantum leap. Human/ET interface and the arrival of a new species or kingdom on Earth." (Jon King)

- "In 2012, Earth's axis will tilt, along with a polar reversal, causing terrestrial and celestial grids to realign, the pineal eye will perceive beyond ultraviolet, and we all ascend to the next dimension beyond time." (Moira Timms)

- "The human race will unify as a single circuit. Solar and galactic sound transmissions will inundate the planetary field. A current charging both poles will race across the skies connecting the polar auroras in a single brilliant flash." (Jose Arguelles)

- "...a moment of quantum awakening. A nanosecond will be stretched into infinity and become non-time, during which we will all experience full consciousness of who we are and why we have incarnated. If we choose to return to human form, we will do so in an awakened state, as reflective cells of the star maker." (Ken Carey)

III. Yes

We are collectively harnessed, by a socialized paradigm or buffer, to the immensity of life in the Universe. Slowly, this is ebbing amidst an evolution of accessible energy, resulting in a myriad of blocked conditions and, hopefully, a resultant process unfolding, called the Spiritual Emergence phenomenon.

It is of necessity that we culturally grock the energetic unification of all life in order to shepherd into reality the next phase of our collective cosmic existence. (It is not unlike the prophetic works of Pierre Teilhard de Chardin and the evolution of Ultra Hominization, enlivening of the Noosphere, the psychic link between brothers and sisters evolving on the heels of the Internet, global communication, and the energy of spherical compression.)

The time is now. The united energy has been increasingly amplified on many planes by the aforementioned Chreode Blazers amidst the two blooms of axial energy: 450-600 B.C. and 1855-1955 A.D. We, the actors, are responding to our lines as the polarity of light expands and nurtures the brothers and sisters who are drawing on lifetimes of experiences to support the qualitative unification of life and its columns of compassion and love. The web has been cast and the pulsing of intuitive connectivity is the message via the proaction of attention and allowance.

Definitively, the relationship that matters is the relationship between the individual and Spirit. Once the relationship is established, the pattern shifts. For it is being attentive to the new pattern that allows the cosmic chiropractic to hold.

Boundaries can be psychically observed until the dimensional door of the pathway opens and one attentively passes with Spirit through to a boundary-free world. Energetic, polarized light composites have been forming as focalizers: Alternative energy, right-livelihood business, green politics, organic food, energy medicine, greenhouse catastrophisms, ET DNA research, the Iraq War, fossil fuel depletion, and Spiritual Emergence have been fed and activated by many of the Chreode Blazers of the two energy pulses.

These have stimulated conscionable consensus as an evolving stage toward unity and a quickening dimensional shift in reality. This cycle of time presages the eminence of planetary transformation and the divine appointment of humankind.

Welcome to the Spirit and Passion of Love.

"Darest though now O soul walk out with me toward the unknown region, where neither ground is for the feet nor any path to follow." — Walt Whitman

Chart A

Earths 7 Planetary Cycles

Saturn

Vulcan

Sun

Venus

Moon

Jupiter

Hyperborean

Earth

India

Atlantis

Present
Greek/Latin

Chart B

7 Major Earth Cycles

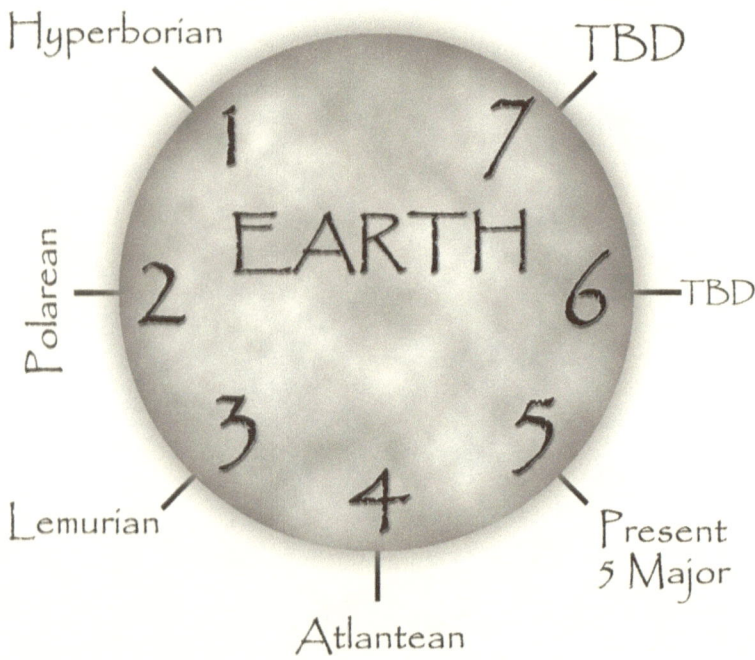

Chart C

7 Minor Cycles In Post Atlantean Cycle

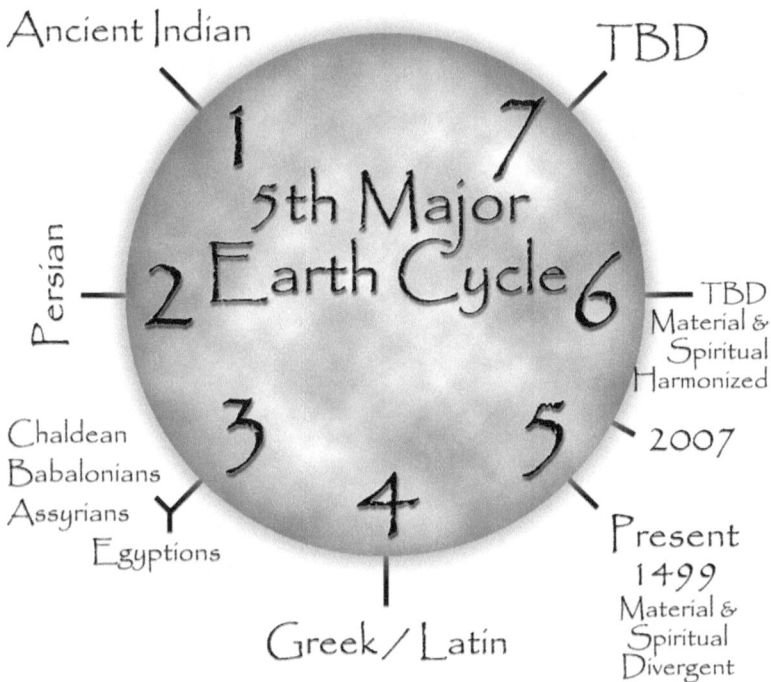

Chart D

24,000 Year Yuga Cycle

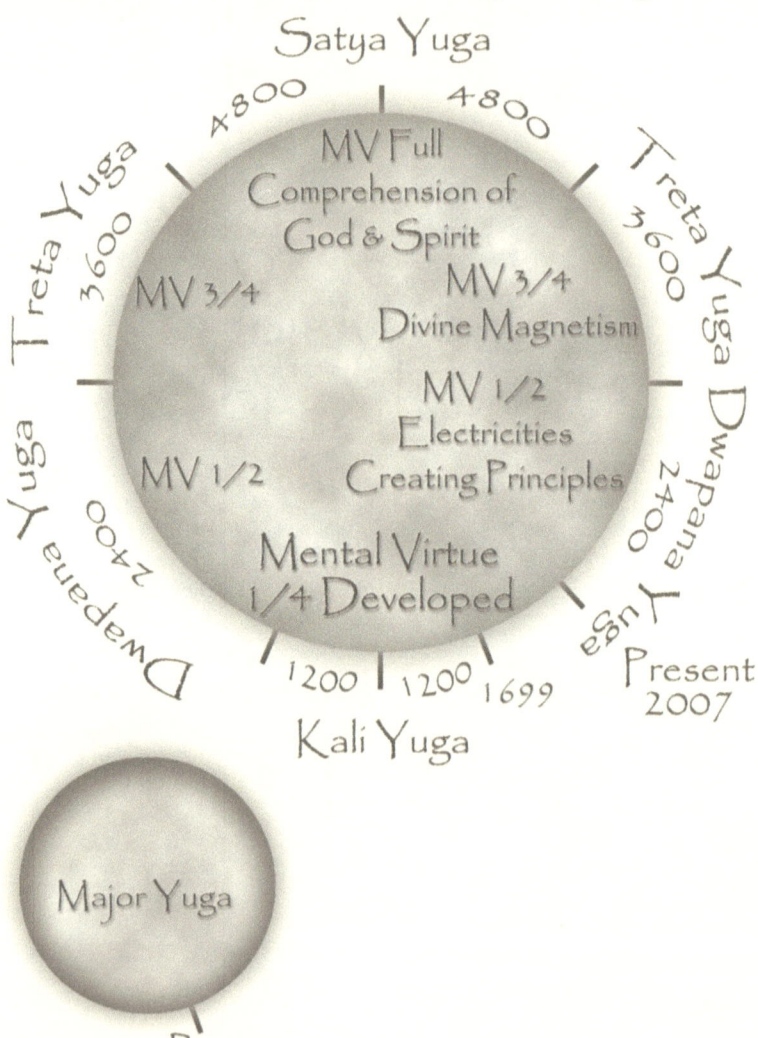

Satya Yuga

Treta Yuga

4,800

4,800

Treta Yuga

3,600

3,600

MV Full
Comprehension of
God & Spirit

MV 3/4

MV 3/4
Divine Magnetism

MV 1/2
Electricities
Creating Principles

MV 1/2

Dwapana Yuga

2,400

2,400

Dwapana Yuga

Mental Virtue
1/4 Developed

Present
2007

1200 1200 1699

Kali Yuga

Major Yuga

Present